Be Beautiful!

Complete Guide to Cosmetics and Body Care

Petra Schürmann

HPBooks
A division of Price Stern Sloan, Inc.
360 North La Cienega Boulevard
Los Angeles, California 90048

ISBN: 0-89586-332-4   Library of Congress Catalog Card Number: 84-80517
©1984 HPBooks, Inc.   Printed in U.S.A.
9 8 7 6 5 4 3

Originally published in Germany as *Das GroBe Buch der Kosmetik und Korperflege*
©1981 Naturalis Publishing Co., Munich-Monchengladbach

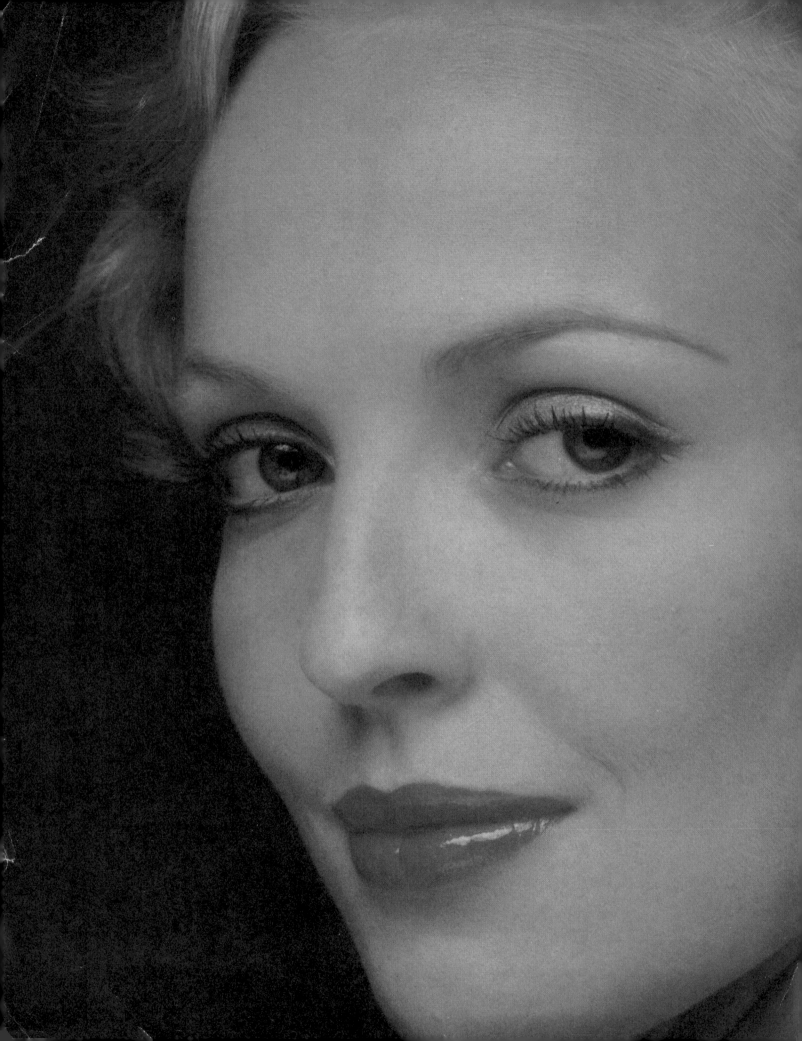

Be Beautiful!

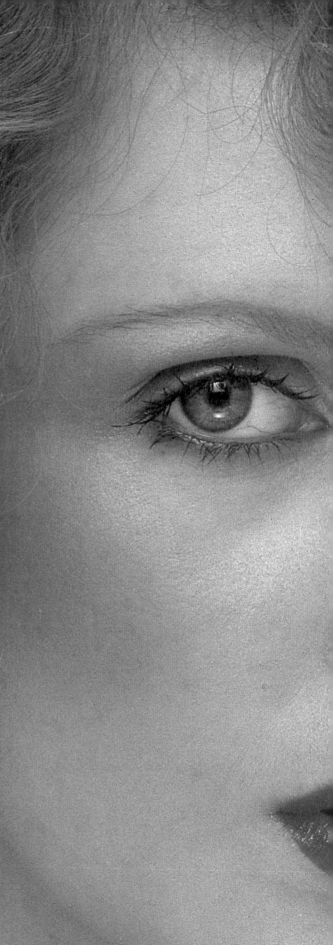

Contents

AMERICAN CONSULTANTS

The publisher would like to thank the following American consultants who reviewed portions of the book:

Karen Beeson, Licensed Cosmetologist and Esthetician
Barbara E. Cox, Pharm.D., R.Ph.
H. Winter Griffith, M.D., Family Medicine
Sue Habkirk, M.A., Instructor in Health Education
Cynthia Hazeltine, M.S., Registered Dietician
Jeff L. Martin, D.D.S., General Dentistry
Kathy Pallija, Herbalist
Charles J. Rolle, M.D., Obstetrician-Gynecologist
Tom Rotkis, M.D., Internal Medicine; Ph.D., Exercise Physiology

Preface

Beauty is an open letter of invitation. It wins even the hearts of strangers, according to the philosopher Schopenhauer. He understood that beauty is the original dream of human beings. No one can resist its effects.

I know that some people disagree with this point of view. They believe these ideas are unfair to people who are not naturally beautiful. They say beauty that must be sustained by artificial means is a masquerade. They say this type of beauty is designed primarily to "catch a man," and women should be too proud to make it an important element in their lives.

I want to say emphatically that I think these people are looking at the concept of beauty in the wrong way.

Every person has something beautiful within herself or himself. Why shouldn't you take care of it? I don't think that hiding little flaws to emphasize your beauty is a masquerade. I see it as an indication that a person is sensitive and aesthetic.

You can't constantly be beautiful for others if you don't want to be beautiful for yourself. Don't you find it slightly depressing to see a sleepy, puffy face in the mirror when you wake up in the morning? Don't you feel fresher and more adventurous when you look at yourself after a little beauty program?

When you like the way you look, you start the day feeling more secure and self-confident. To pretend this isn't true is to deceive yourself.

An entire industry has been built around this idea. Every day corporations compete for our attention with new products designed to make us look better and feel better.

This abundance of products creates its own problems. It has never been so difficult to figure out which cosmetics will be most effective. Many young girls and even older women don't know where to begin. They give up before they start.

It *is* difficult to find the products that will work best for you. The results will never be satisfactory if you try to model yourself after a movie star.

The most important step in making yourself more beautiful is looking at yourself carefully. Note the strengths and weaknesses of your face and body. This is the only way to ensure that you will get the best results from cosmetics.

This book is built on basic beauty principles. It presents the most effective techniques and products for making yourself as lovely as you can be. The book includes techniques and advice for using cosmetics and beauty care products. It is designed to help you become a happier, more confident person, whose looks are a letter of recommendation.

Petra Schürmann

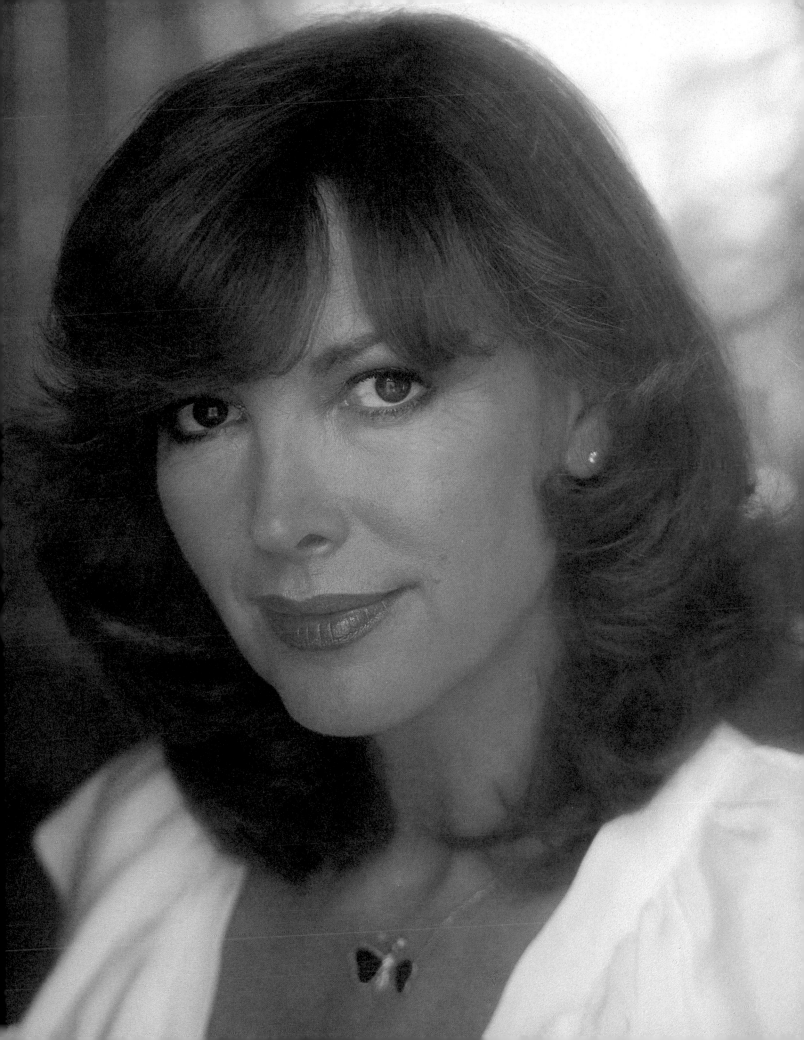

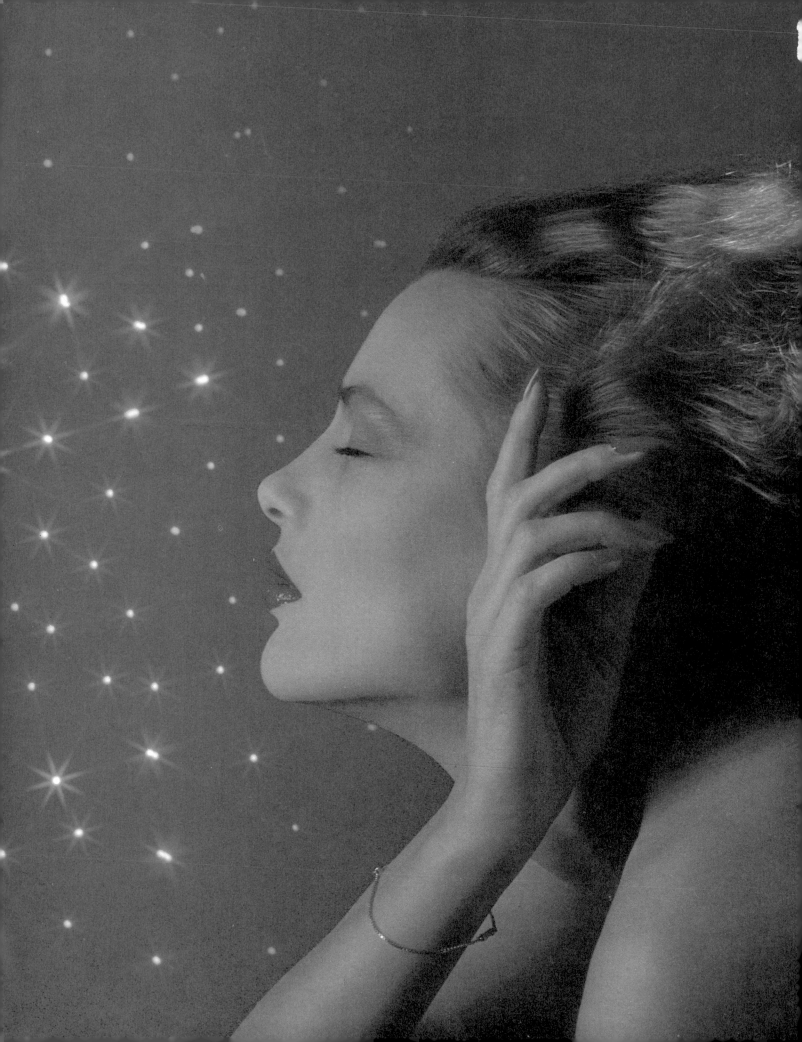

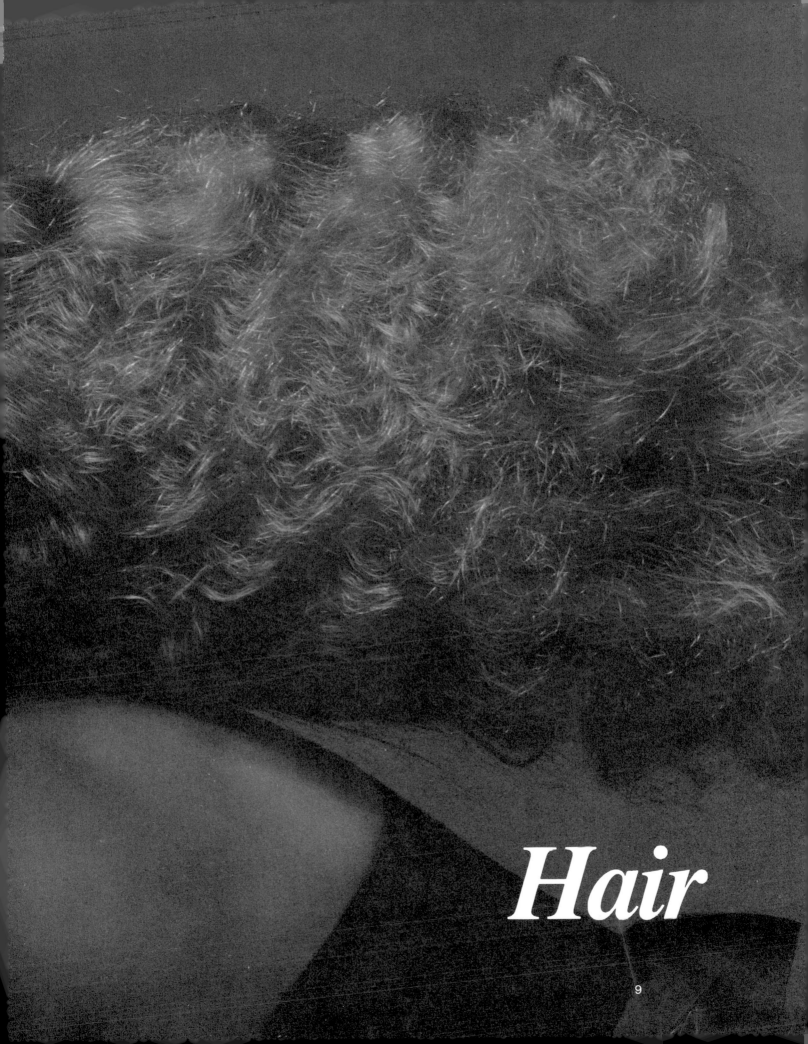

Hair

You may not have thought about it, but your hair is the only part of your body that you can manipulate to your heart's content. You can cut it, grow it, curl or straighten it, color it blond or even green. You can style it one way today and another tomorrow. It can make you look practical, sophisticated or sexy. You can change your hair constantly, on one condition: Your hair must be *healthy*. Only then will it be shiny and clean no matter what you do with it. Maintaining healthy hair is a problem for many women. On the following pages you will find information about care and styling for every hair type.

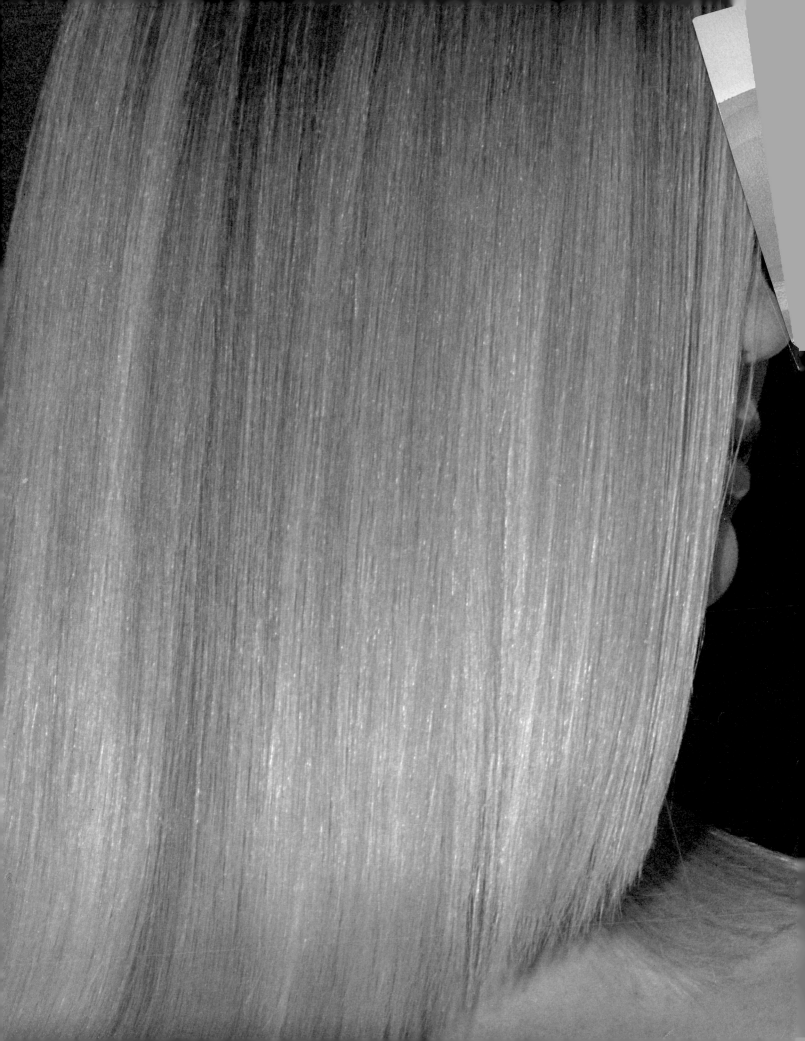

Hair Types

Before you start a hair-care program, you have to know what hair type you have. Is it oily, dry or normal? You also need to examine the condition of your hair. Is it brittle? Does it have split ends?

Oily Hair — Excessive oil occurs when the *sebaceous glands,* the oil glands in the scalp, are overactive. Sometimes this condition is related to hormonal imbalances. Once the scalp becomes greasy, brushing and combing make the entire hair shaft oily. If your hair becomes oily quickly, use special products formulated for oily hair.

Dry Hair — Dryness is caused by underactive sebaceous glands. However, dry hair can also be caused by stress, too much sun, using a blow dryer at high settings or brushing hair too frequently or vigorously. Dry hair frequently leads to split ends and hair breakage, because not enough oil is distributed over the hair shaft.

Fine Hair — Fine hair has shafts that are thinner than normal. Fine hair can be either oily or dry. It is very sensitive and easily damaged by harsh hair-care products and the sun.

Dandruff — Numerous factors, including bacteria and fungus, can cause dandruff. This problem can occur when a scalp is extremely oily or extremely dry. Dandruff is aggravated if the scalp is not thoroughly rinsed after shampooing or conditioning. You can control dandruff with special shampoos, but you can't cure it. Brushing your hair and scalp with a natural-bristle brush before shampooing loosens flakes so your scalp can be cleansed more thoroughly.

Split Ends—These occur because hair ends endure months of washing, combing and exposure to the elements. Braiding your hair can cause split ends. Using permanents and rollers can also split your hair. After an end splits, the entire shaft may break. Hair looks brittle, dull and uneven.

Damaged Hair—Hair in this condition feels rough and brittle. It is also unmanageable. Damage occurs when the protective outer layer of the hair shaft is worn away by chemicals or excessive exposure to the elements.

Damaged hair can contribute to hair loss.

Hair Loss—Everyone loses approximately 80 to 100 hairs every day. If you think you are losing more than that, consult a dermatologist. Many factors contribute to hair loss, including illness, medication, and hormonal or metabolic imbalances. It can also be an inherited trait.

Sun, wind and rain can damage your hair.

13

Washing Hair

Beautiful hair requires proper care. This starts with shampooing. Make sure your shampoo is appropriate for your hair type and is pH-balanced. The label should say, "pH-balanced" or "acid-balanced."

Oily-hair shampoos have ingredients to gently cleanse the scalp and slow the production of oil by the sebaceous glands.

Dandruff shampoos contain bacteria-killing substances.

Dry-hair shampoos have moisturizers, and those for damaged hair contain conditioners. Although shampoos for dry and damaged hair are very mild, you can't rely solely on these shampoos to restore your hair. You must also use conditioners.

Fine-hair shampoos contain substances that give hair more body.

You should wash your hair as soon as it looks oily, limp or unmanageable. Most people need to wash their hair every day.

If you have long hair, brush it vigorously and make sure all tangles are gone before you wash it.

Wet your hair thoroughly before you shampoo. Never apply shampoo directly to your hair. Put a small amount in the palm of your hand and add a little water. Then apply the shampoo to your hair and gently massage the scalp with your fingertips. You don't need a great deal of shampoo to clean your hair. Most shampoos are concentrated, so it's better to use less.

Wet hair swells and is more susceptible to damage, so never pull your hair while shampooing.

Let shampoo stay in your hair approximately 30 seconds. Rinse your hair thoroughly. If you don't rinse out all the shampoo and conditioners, your hair will be sticky and dull. Hair is completely clean if it squeaks when you run your fingers along the shaft.

Be sure to use a pH-balanced shampoo. Others contain harsh detergents that can damage your hair.

Water temperature is important when you shampoo and rinse. If water is too hot, it activates the sebaceous glands, causing hair to become oily more quickly. If the final rinse water is cold, it gives hair a nice shine and improves circulation to the scalp.

Always be sure to use fresh towels. Bacteria can be transferred from towels to the scalp. This can lead to dandruff and other types of scalp irritation.

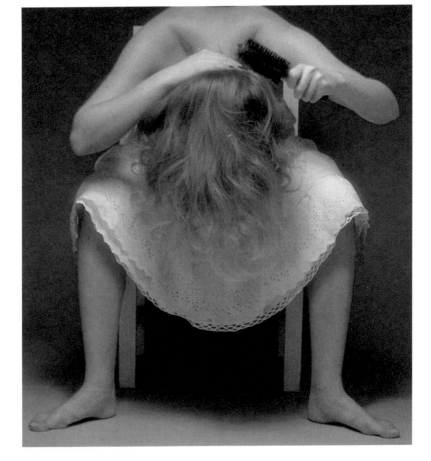

Proper hair care begins with shampooing. Brush hair well before applying shampoo.

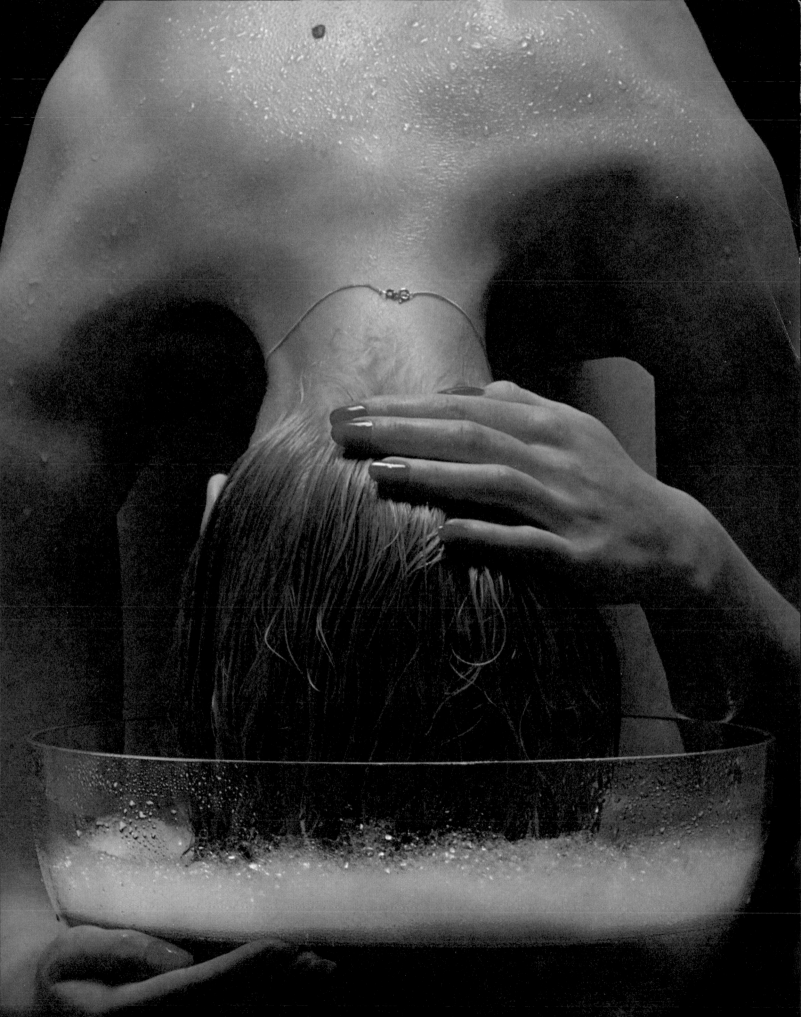

Conditioners and Rinses

Conditioners and creme rinses give hair more sheen. Rinses untangle and smooth the surface of the hair, which helps prevent damage.

Conditioners assist in restoring hair. However, if your hair is severely damaged, no product can completely restore it. Your hair will have to be cut.

Use a creme rinse after every wash. Use a conditioner every third or fourth wash.

For dry hair, apply creme rinse to the hair and scalp. For normal hair, apply rinse to the hair only. For oily hair, apply rinse to the ends only. You can rinse out most creme rinses after 60 seconds.

Use creme rinse after every shampoo to protect and untangle your hair.

Sometimes homemade rinses can give oily hair more shine. Try adding 1 tablespoon of lemon juice and a dash of vinegar to 1 pint of water (2 cups). Alternate this rinse with your creme rinse.

Using conditioners regularly will keep your hair healthy and will alleviate some scalp problems.

Be sure to get conditioners designed for your hair type or problem. For example, it would be a mistake to use conditioners for damaged hair on soft, fine hair. These conditioners contain softeners, which fine hair doesn't need.

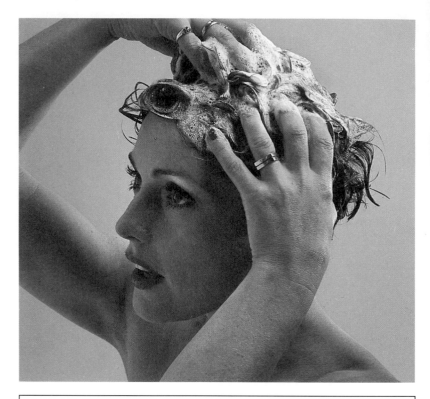

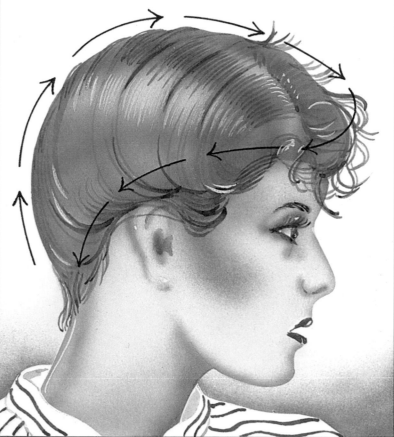

Apply all conditioners according to directions. Be sure to work them gently into the hair with your fingertips, then comb them through. You can intensify the effects of conditioners by applying heat. Put a plastic bag or plastic wrap over your hair to hold in body heat. Using a blow dryer or hood dryer is even more effective.

Cosmetologists can help you plan your hair-care program. They can examine your hair and scalp and diagnose any problems. For example, you may have an oily scalp, but dry hair.

Nearly every beauty salon carries a full line of hair-care products. A cosmetologist can choose the best conditioner for you and show you how to use it at home.

Comb wet hair only after you have applied the conditioner or creme rinse.

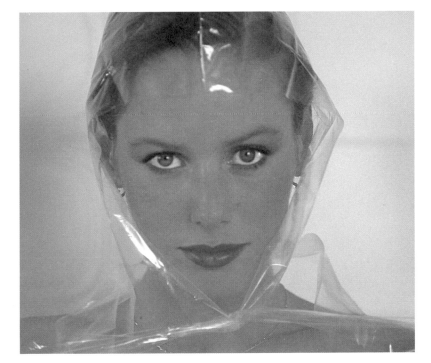

Conditioners for fine, dry or damaged hair should be worked gently into the hair, then combed through with a wide-tooth comb.

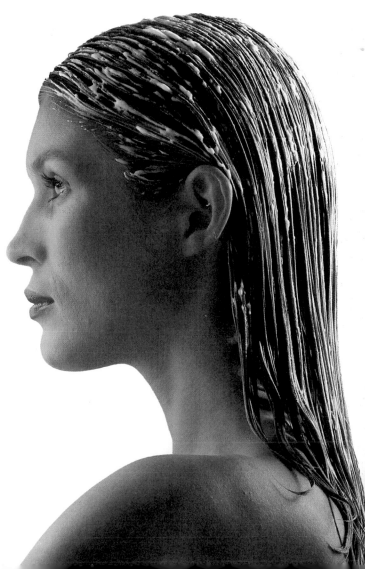

Choosing the Right Tools

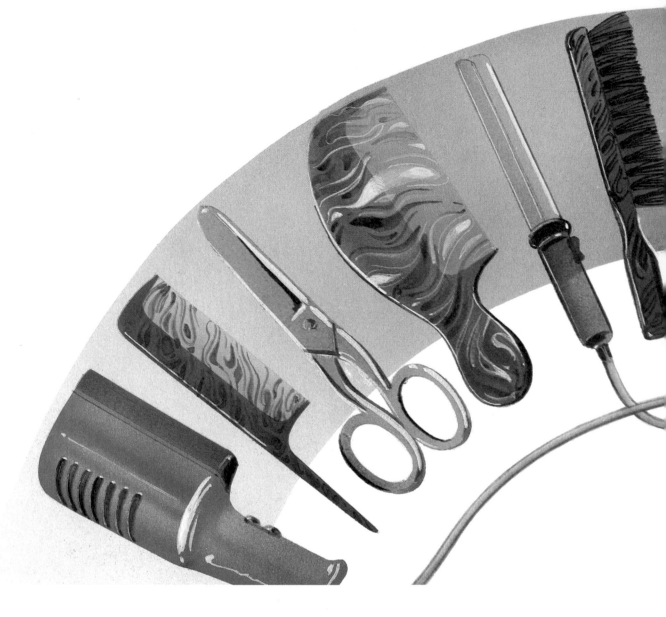

Beautiful, healthy hair is more important to your appearance than the most extravagant dress. To keep hair looking its best, you must use the proper equipment. Using the wrong brush or comb can irritate the scalp, spread dandruff and damage hair. Quality equipment is expensive, but it contributes greatly to the health of your hair.

Combs are especially important. Large combs with wide teeth work best. Smaller combs tend to snag, which can split and break the hair shaft. Extra-large combs or picks, called *Afro combs,* are ideal for hair that is permed, colored or tightly curled.

Good combs come in different materials. Tortoise-shell and horn combs are the most beautiful, but they are expensive. Hard rubber combs work just as well and are much less expensive.

Use coated rubber bands for ponytails. Ordinary rubber bands will break your hair.

Brushes are also essential to good hair care. The best

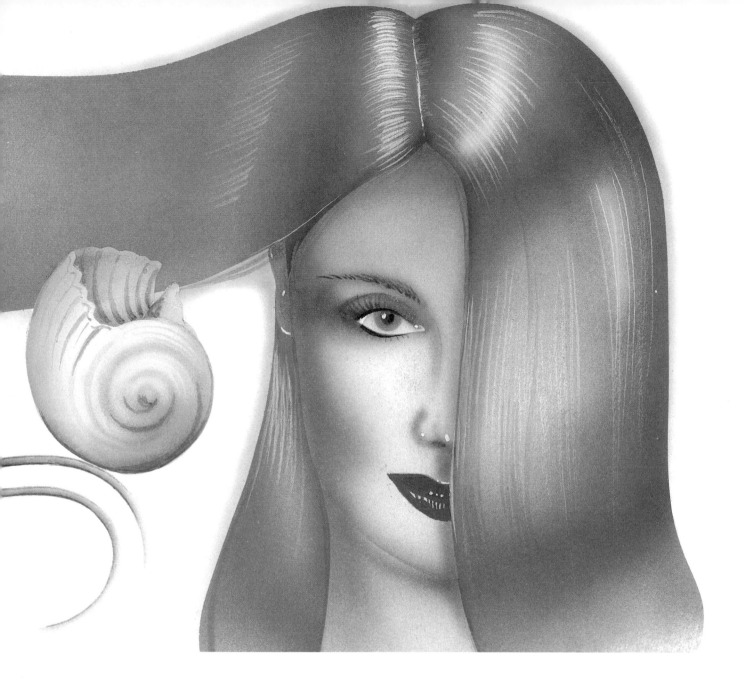

brushes are those with flexible bristles.

Test bristles by running your fingers over them. If they sting or feel stiff, they could damage your hair.

If you don't use a brush to style your hair, buy one with natural bristles. If you do use a brush with your blow dryer, buy one with widely separated plastic bristles. Bristles on the best styling brushes have rounded tips. Styling brushes with bristles that go all the way around the head of the brush are the most effective. Remember, the smaller the brush, the tighter the curl.

Rollers should also be purchased carefully. Buy smooth ones. Those with bristles or sharp protrusions can break your hair.

Remember that steam curling irons are harder on hair than other types. They produce more heat and can severely damage your hair.

High-quality combs, brushes and appliances are indispensible.

Blow-Drying Your Hair

Blow-dried hairstyles look soft and natural. However, you may find you can't style your hair as beautifully as a cosmetologist can. If this is the case, you are making one of three mistakes: Your hair is too wet when you start drying it, you stop drying too soon or you aren't parting your hair properly.

Blow-drying will be easier and your style more beautiful if you follow these suggestions: After rinsing your hair, towel-dry it thoroughly. Then wet it with a blow-dry lotion. This gives hair more body and helps the comb or brush glide through it more easily. Bend from the waist and let your hair fall forward. Hold the dryer parallel to your hair, about 6 inches away. Turn on the dryer and move it continually until hair is 90% dry.

Straighten up, comb and part your hair, then finish blow-drying. Start with your bangs, using your brush to provide direction and curl.

Then dry the sides of your hair one section at a time. Each section should be as wide as the head of the brush. Take each section and brush it through. Then place the hair ends flat on the brush. Roll the brush under for a pageboy, up for a flip. The tighter you roll the brush, the tighter the curl. As you dry each section, move the dryer constantly.

If you have thick, wavy hair and want a natural style, move the dryer randomly while mussing hair with your fingers. Just before your hair is dry, use a brush to style it.

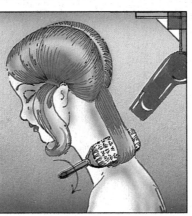

If your hair curls when it rains, use setting lotion. It helps keep moisture out of your hair.

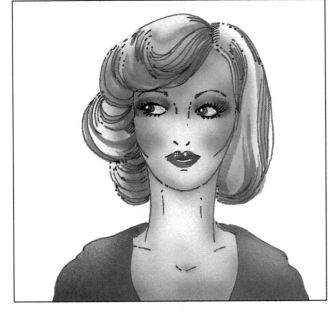

To style your hair, part it in sections. Curl each section around your brush. The smaller the section and brush, the tighter the curl.

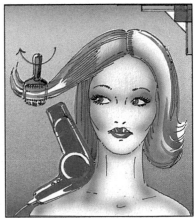

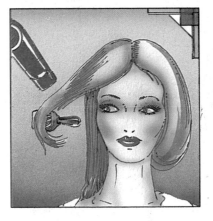

Rolling Techniques

Rolling hair properly isn't an art. It's a matter of practice.

Be sure to use plastic rollers or rollers covered with foam rubber. They are much easier on your hair.

Your hairstyle will last longer if you use setting lotion. This product contains water, alcohol and artificial resin. It forms a fine film around your hair, which strengthens and protects the shaft. Setting lotions for oily hair act like blotting paper. They absorb excess oil. Setting lotions for dry hair contain moisturizers. Those for damaged hair contain substances that make hair smoother and more manageable. All setting lotions give hair more body.

Obstinate ends are hard to handle at first. If they are not lying flat, they will bend or break. Don't be discouraged. Practice makes perfect.

Picture 1
Start the rolling process by making a part on each side of one section of hair at the top of your head. The easiest way to do this is to use the long, pointed handle of a rat-tail comb. Be sure the section isn't too thick, or it will take too long to dry.

Pull the section straight up and comb it through.

Picture 2
Hold the section straight and put the hair ends flat on the roller. If the ends are dry, moisten them slightly.

Picture 3
Turn the roller slowly and carefully. Roll your hair tightly, but don't pull it so hard that you feel the pull in your scalp.

Picture 4
Keep one finger on the roller to prevent the hair from slipping off. Keep turning the roller until it reaches the scalp. It should lie in the center of the two parts you made.

Picture 5
Secure the roller with a clip. Insert the clip at an angle, so it lies flat on the scalp. Roll the rest of your hair, section by section, in the same manner.

Remove rollers only when your hair is completely dry and cool.

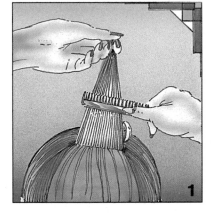

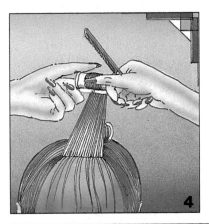

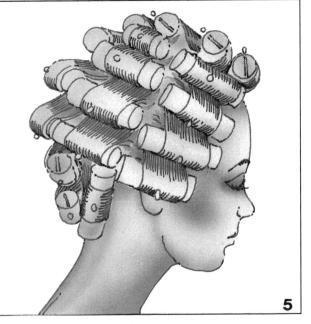

Electric Rollers

Electric rollers come in kits of 10 to 20. Each roller has its own heating element. The number and size you will need will depend on your hairstyle.

Don't put electric rollers in wet hair. It is too fragile. Blow-dry your hair first.

Heat the electric rollers for 15 minutes. Then use the techniques recommended on page 21.

Use large rollers for hair at the top of your head, and smaller ones for hair on the sides and back.

Take time to roll your hair neatly on the rollers. The more careful you are, the easier it will be to remove the rollers.

Unroll rollers when they have cooled completely. Let hair cool 5 minutes before brushing or combing it.

Using electric rollers too often can damage and split your hair. Once this happens, hair must be trimmed to prevent further damage.

Cosmetologists do this by twisting hair tight, one small section at a time. This makes the broken parts of each shaft stick out. They can then be cut.

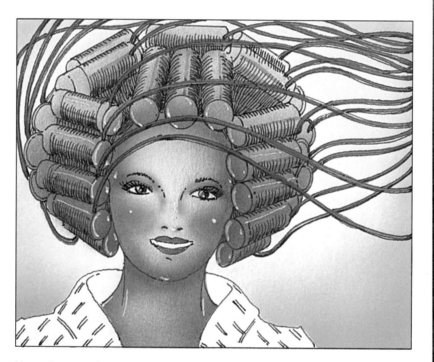

Use rollers carefully to minimize damage to your hair.

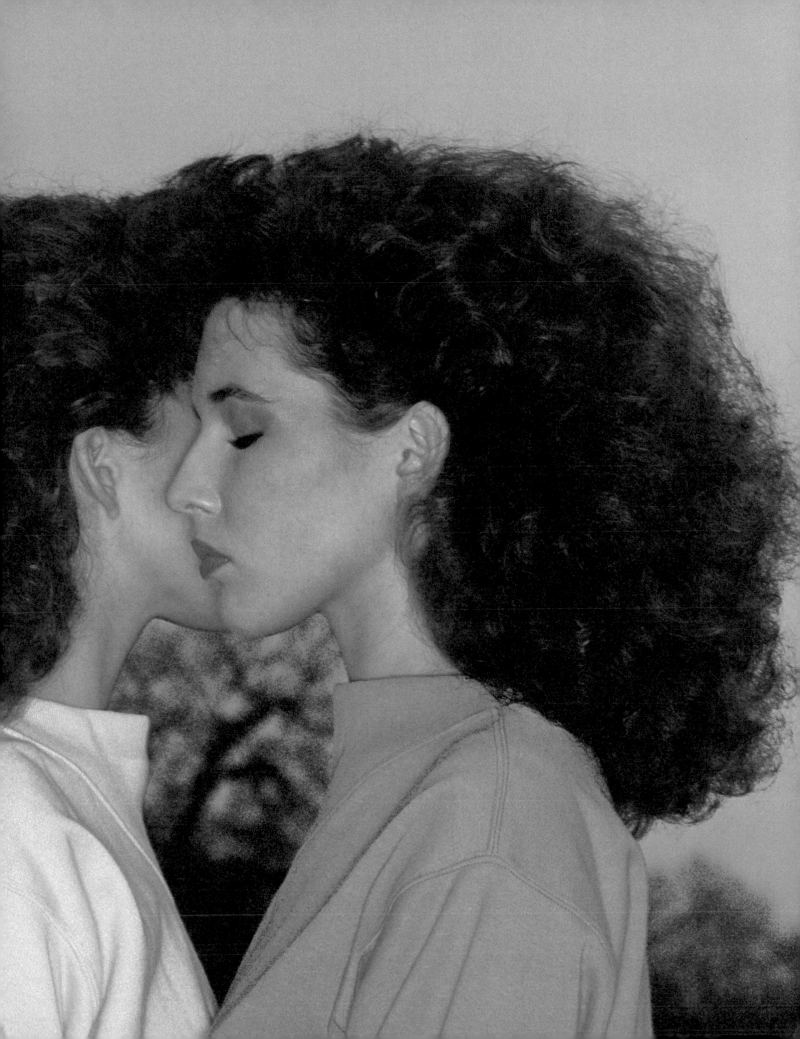

Curling and Waving Techniques

If you want curls that last weeks or months, get a permanent. If you want curls only occasionally, you may use one of seven techniques. Each is less harsh than a perm, and its effects disappear with your next shampoo.

Bobby Pins—You can obtain soft waves by rolling your hair around your finger and securing the curl with bobby pins. You need approximately two packages of bobby pins. Start with the hair at the top of your head. Take a small section of hair. Run the comb through it to ensure that no tangles are present. Starting at the scalp, gently wind the hair in the direction you want the wave to go. After forming the curl, secure it to the scalp with a bobby pin.

Don't apply setting lotion. It makes hair frizzy when used with bobby pins.

Clips—This technique is suitable only for short or medium-length hair. Roll the hair as you would for bobby pins and clip in place. If you have fine hair, you can apply a little setting lotion beforehand.

For best results, put a hairnet over the curls and let them dry naturally.

Rollers—These work best if you have long hair and want a loose, wavy style. Be sure to use setting lotion. Follow the suggestions on page 21 about rolling techniques.

Perm Rods—These produce tight, natural-looking waves. Take a small section of hair by the ends. Comb until completely smooth. Place a piece of tissue paper around the

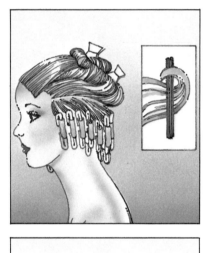

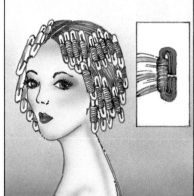

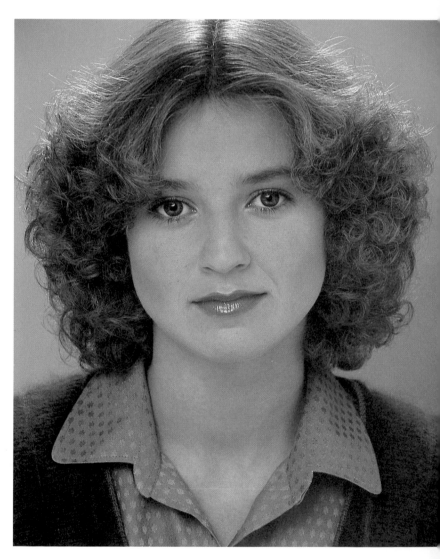

hair ends. Then wrap them around the bottom of the perm rod. Roll the rod up until it reaches the scalp. Close the top of the rod to hold your hair in place.

Braids—This technique takes a lot of time. Be sure your hair is very damp, and apply setting lotion before you start.

Take a small section of hair and begin braiding at the scalp. Braid all the way to the ends. The tighter the braid, the tighter the curl.

Before you have a perm, experiment with different hairstyles.

Curling Iron—This is good for touch-ups. Be sure to put hair ends flat on the iron. Close the iron and roll it to the scalp. The longer you keep your hair wrapped around the iron, the tighter the curl will be.

Crimping Iron—Crimped curls give your hairstyle a youthful look. You don't have to crimp all your hair. A style may look better if you crimp only a few strands. To use the crimping iron, start at the scalp, close the iron for a few seconds, then open it. Continue in this manner down the hair strand. Curls last 2 to 3 days.

Blow-dry your hair for a few minutes if you use small rollers. Otherwise, your hair will take too long to dry.

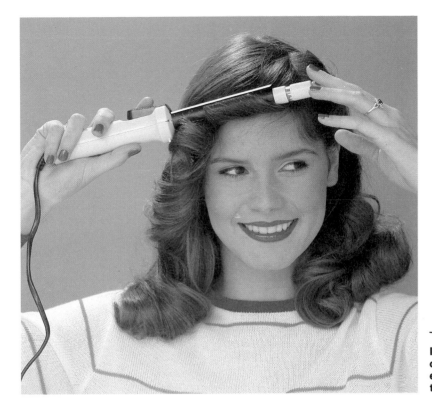

If you want curls only occasionally, you can experiment with the seven techniques listed at left.

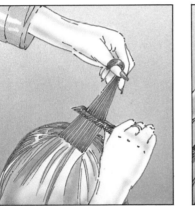 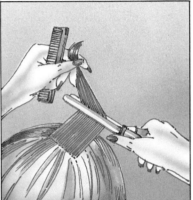

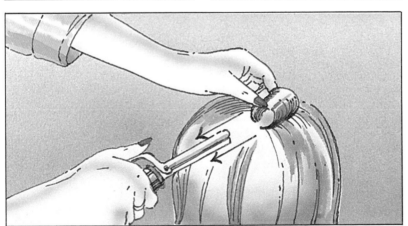

Styling Tips for Fine Hair

The most effective way to make fine hair appear thicker is to choose the right hairstyle. The best styles are short, blunt and built around a good scissor-cut. Resign yourself to the fact that many other styles simply will not work. Your hair will not be able to hold them. If you continue to try wearing these styles, you'll only be unhappy and less attractive than you should be.

Giving your hair a color treatment or permanent can sometimes add body. The reason is that if you have fine hair, each shaft has an abnormally smooth surface. Each layer lies perfectly flat.

Use only setting lotions made especially for fine hair. They put a protective film around each strand, giving hair more body and strength.

Careful teasing and blow-drying make your hairstyle last longer.

Proper drying techniques also create more body. With all hairstyles except perms, blow-drying hair in the opposite direction from the way it will be styled makes hair look fuller. Lean forward from the waist and let your hair fall

Holding the dryer 6 inches from your hair, dry the section thoroughly. For a long-lasting style, leave the brush in place until your hair is cool.

Teasing has become popular again. This technique is not good for your hair, but it won't do any lasting damage if you only use it occasionally.

Teasing gives fine, soft hair more fullness. Tease hair from the scalp to the middle of the strand. Never tease all the way to the end of the strand.

Tease only hair that will give your style the body and lift you want. With short styles this may be a few strands or a very small section in the crown area.

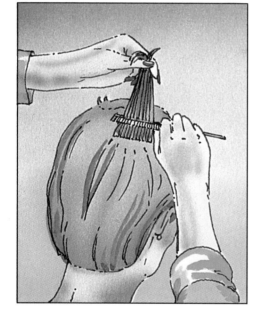

Teasing fine hair gives it more body. Always tease gently, so your hair doesn't look like a nest.

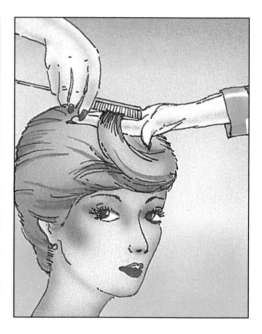

Color and perm preparations contain chemicals that make the shaft thicker and more uneven. Hair looks fuller and holds curls and waves longer.

Fine hair must always look dainty, so wash it often. Use shampoos formulated to give your hair extra body.

Apply setting lotions sparingly. If you use too much, hair will look stiff and lifeless.

forward. Hold the dryer 6 inches from your hair and move it continually from the neck to the top of the scalp.

When your hair is almost dry, straighten up and begin styling. Make a part on each side of one section of hair. Put the ends of the hair flat on your round styling brush. Gently turn the brush in the direction you want the curl to go.

Because fine hair is thin and fragile, you must choose hair-care equipment carefully. Use only soft-bristle brushes and wide-tooth combs. Make sure your dryer has several temperature settings and never use the hot setting. Use electric rollers, curling irons and similar devices only occasionally. They can easily damage fine hair.

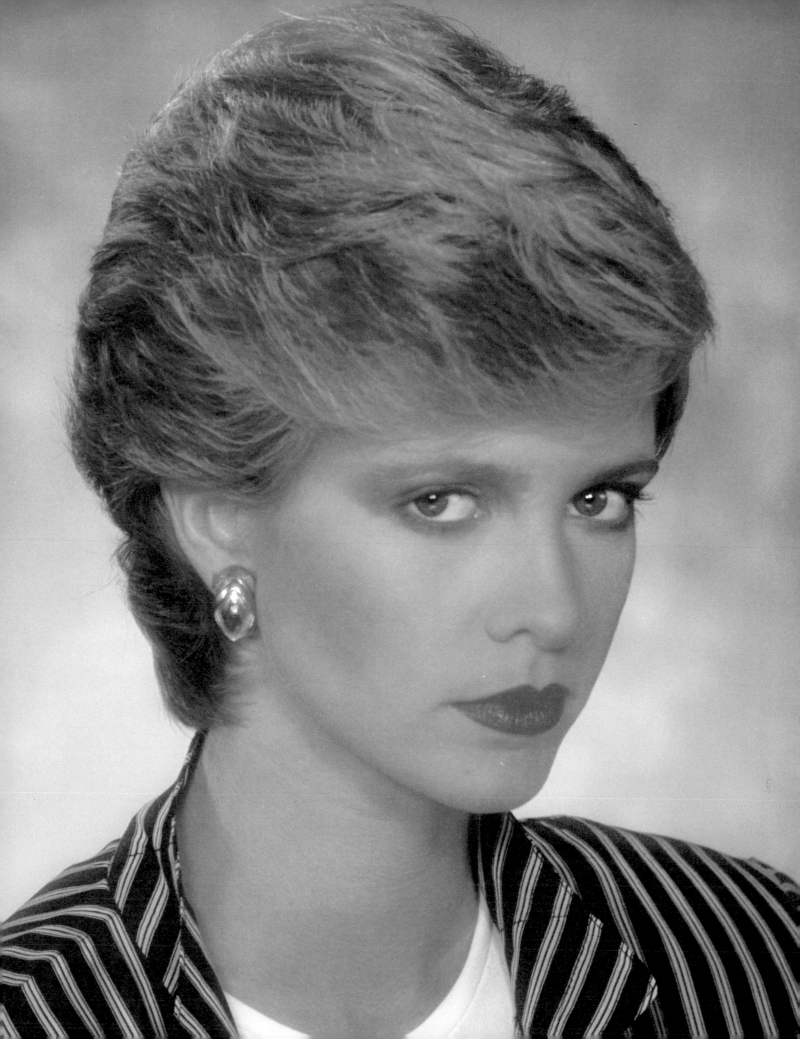

Choosing the Best Hairstyle

Your facial type determines which hairstyle is the most flattering. The four major types are *oval, heart-shaped, rectangular* and *round*. You can determine what type you have by pulling back your hair and tracing the outline of your face on a mirror with crayon.

Remember that the best hairstyles have several common characteristics. They have a classic look, so you can wear them for years. You don't have to change your hair with every new fashion trend. These styles are also easy to care for. You can do everything yourself. The only thing you'll

need from a beauty salon is a good, basic haircut.

The most ideal face type is oval. Almost any hairstyle is flattering, especially if it frames the face. Short, layered styles are pretty, with or without

---

Unhappy with the shape of your face? You can minimize its flaws by choosing an appropriate hairstyle.

---

bangs. The sides should fall gently away from the part and cover the ears. Long hair with

soft waves or curls looks very sensual. It should reach just below the shoulders.

A heart-shaped face also looks beautiful with almost any hairstyle. Some people with this facial type have a chin that is a little too pointed, but this is easy to minimize.

The best short styles have a long top layer. The front of this layer is brushed in a wave across the forehead. The side layers are brushed back. The back of the hair is kept very full.

Long, straight hair looks good in a Mona Lisa style. Hair is parted in the center. Ends can be curled into a pageboy or

Is your face oval, heart-shaped, rectangular or round? These are the four major facial types.

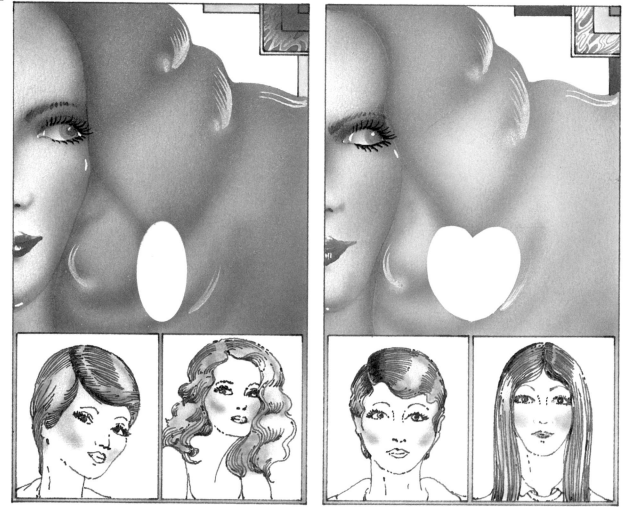

flip. If you want to keep this style indefinitely, give the ends a perm. This will give the style more body.

If you have a rectangular face, you need a hairstyle that makes its contours appear shorter and wider. This means you should not wear long, straight hair or styles parted in the middle. They will make your face look more elongated.

If you have medium-length or long hair, try a hairstyle that is full at the sides and frames your face. Bangs that sweep across the forehead are also flattering.

If you want a short, curly style, part the hair at the side and roll the hair on lots of rollers to add fullness. If you have naturally curly hair or a perm, cut your hair to chin length.

You can see what facial type you have by pulling back your hair and outlining the contours of your face on a mirror with crayon.

People used to think that if you had a round face, you could only wear two or three hairstyles. Today we know better. If you have a round face you can wear numerous styles.

If you have short hair and want a curly style, be sure it has plenty of bounce. Thin, short bangs can also make your face look less chubby. If you want a smoother style, get a layered cut and comb the hair away from the face.

Long hair can look very elegant. It should be blunt-cut at shoulder length and worn in a soft pageboy. Bangs that sweep to one side make this style even more becoming.

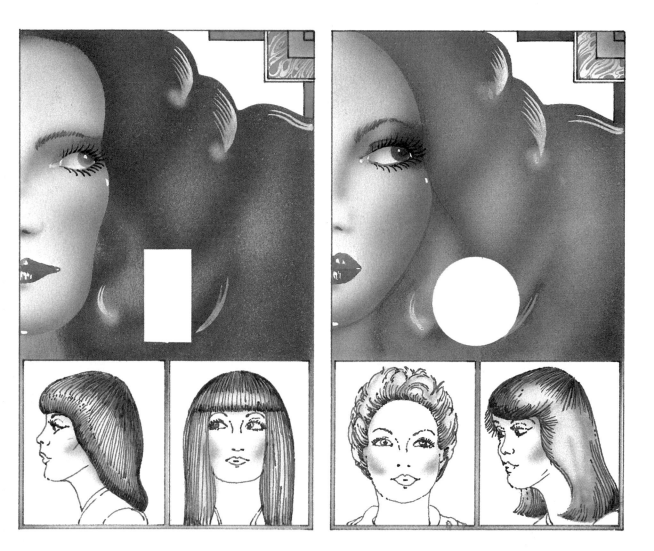

Hair-Coloring Tips

Hair color is important with simple, straight hairstyles. You don't have to be unhappy with your hair color. New products make it easy to give your hair interesting highlights or to turn it a different shade entirely.

Before you decide to change your hair color, be sure you know the difference between *permanent* and *semipermanent* colors.

Permanent hair colors, or tints, penetrate and chemically alter the hair shaft. They reduce natural pigments and add artificial ones. The lighter the new color, the stronger the preparation. Because the chemicals involved are so harsh, hair that has been colored must be groomed very carefully.

Semipermanent hair colors do not penetrate the hair shaft. Pigment is laid on the surface of the shaft and color develops though oxidation. Semipermanent hair colors darken hair and add natural-looking highlights. They cannot be used to lighten hair.

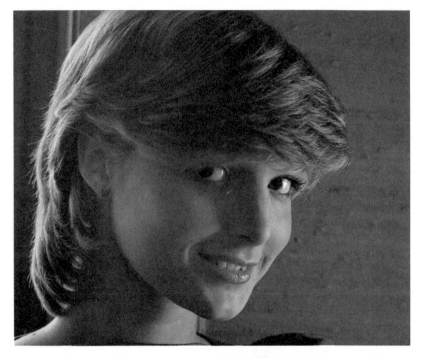

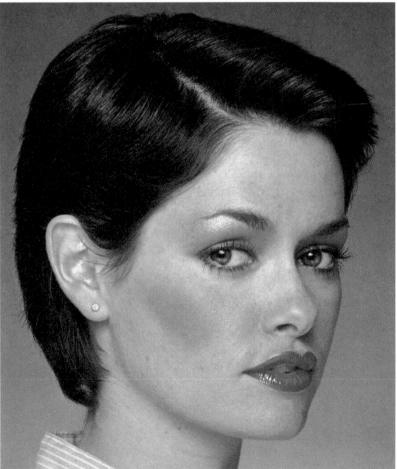

Using color makes short hair look more lively. The hairstyle in the photo at right can be worn with or without bangs.

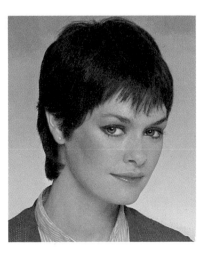

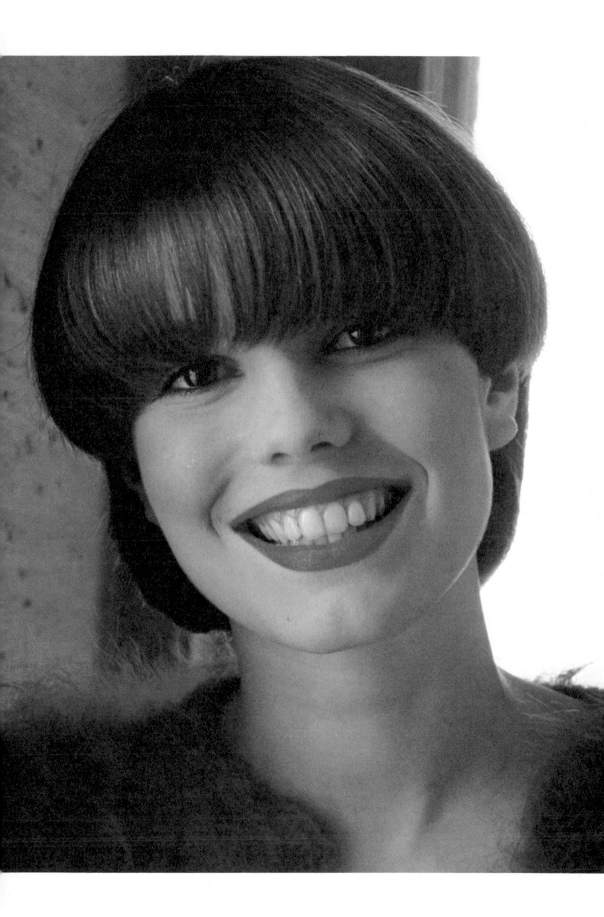

This hairstyle is ideal for short, thin hair. Blow-dry your hair from the scalp down. Use a small brush to give your hair more body.

Highlighting and Sun Streaking

Highlighting and *sun streaking* make hair more beautiful. You should have this done at a beauty salon. New techniques give hair natural-looking highlights instead of a streaked look.

The highlighted parts of your hair should be no more than three shades lighter than the natural color. The darker your natural color, the less difference there should be. If you have ash-blond hair, highlighted strands should be gold-blond, red-blond or both. If you have brown hair, highlighted sections should be auburn or red. Have your hair highlighted every 3 to 4 months.

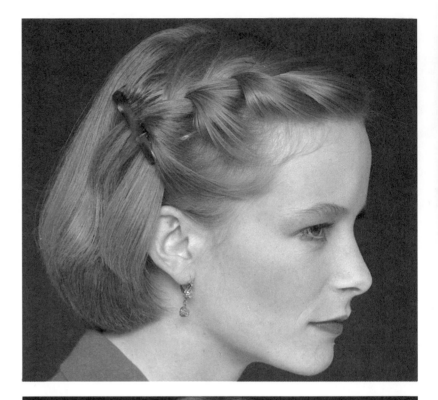

Cosmetologists call this hairstyle a *bob*, below and right. The hair on the sides and in the back is one length. The bangs are straight and full. For variety you can brush back a wide section and pin it with a small comb.

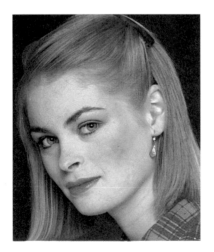

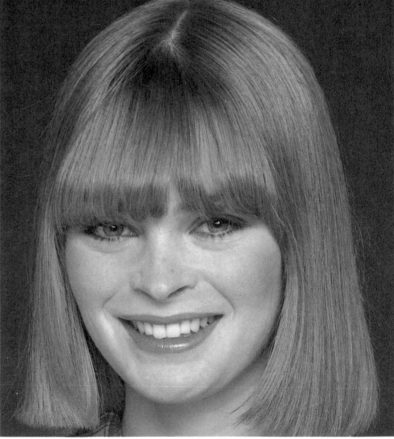

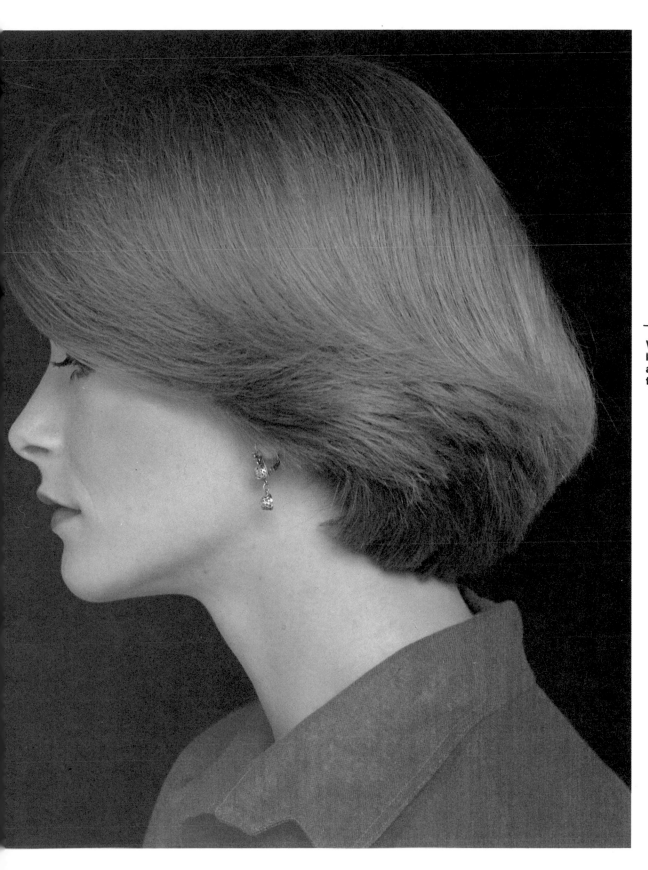

With this style, the hair is layered only at the neck and swings gently away from the side part.

Perming Tips

Permanent waves have been dramatically improved in the past few years. You can get anything from soft, natural-looking curls to a tight Afro look, depending on the rod size used.

Hair must be healthy for a perm to be effective. If your hair has been sun-bleached, or treated with chemicals or henna, call this to the cosmetologist's attention.

Be sure all split ends are trimmed before you get a perm. This ensures that the ends of the hair won't look frizzy.

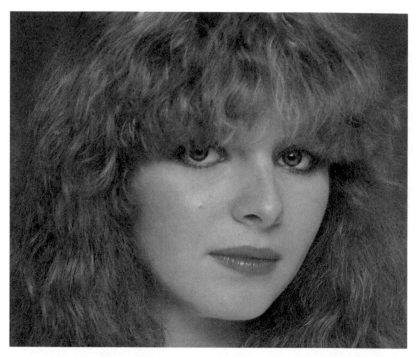

The hairstyle in the upper-right photo is a perm. The style in the lower-right photo looks more natural, despite the artificial curl. Try parting the bangs and pinning the hair into a small chignon.

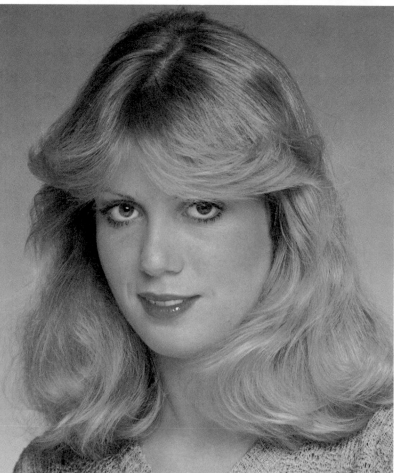

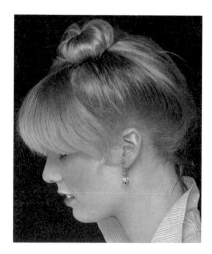

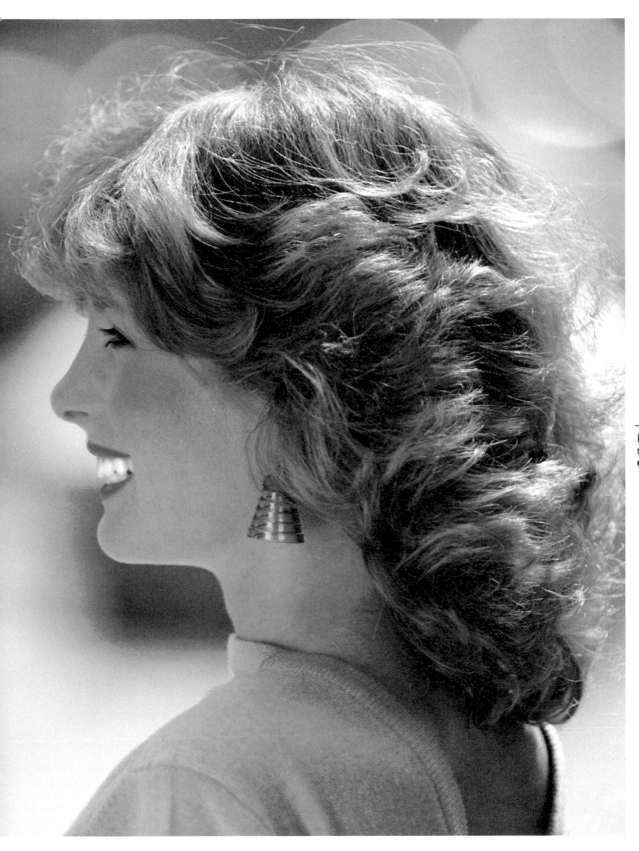

Long hair is beautiful and sexy. If yours doesn't have enough curl, try a perm.

Hairstyles for Evening

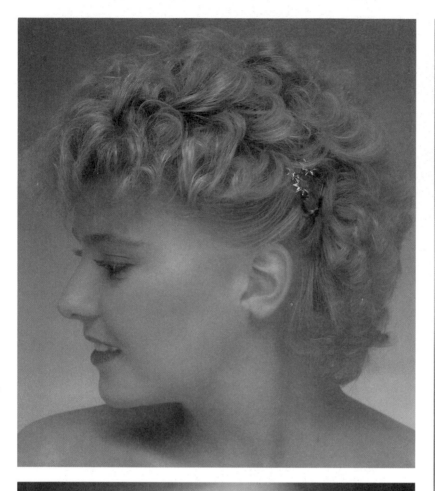

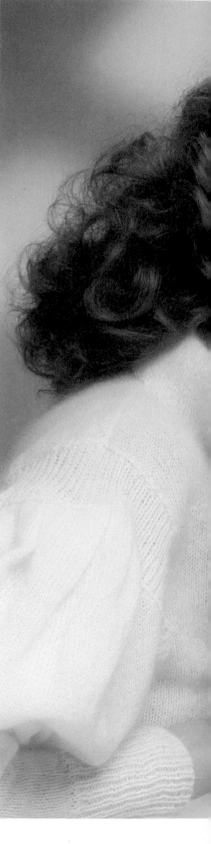

A decorative pin, clip or comb can make a curly style more elegant.

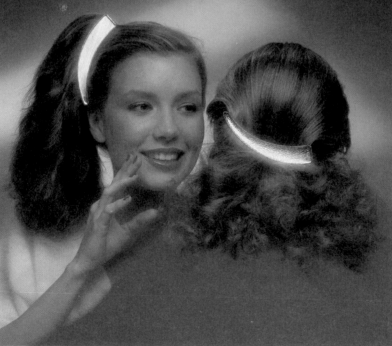

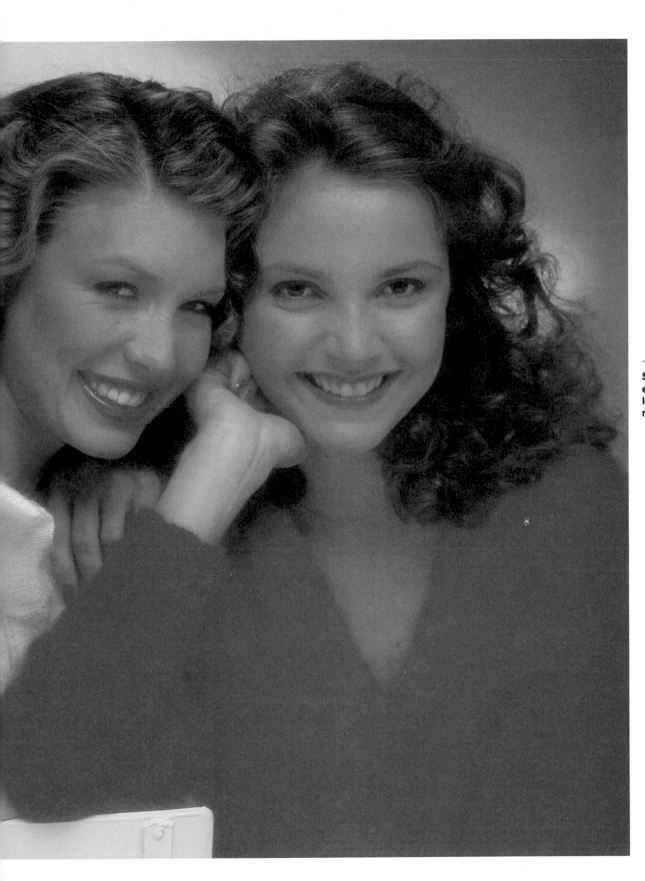

Soft curls look
especially nice with
long hair, but they
require more work.

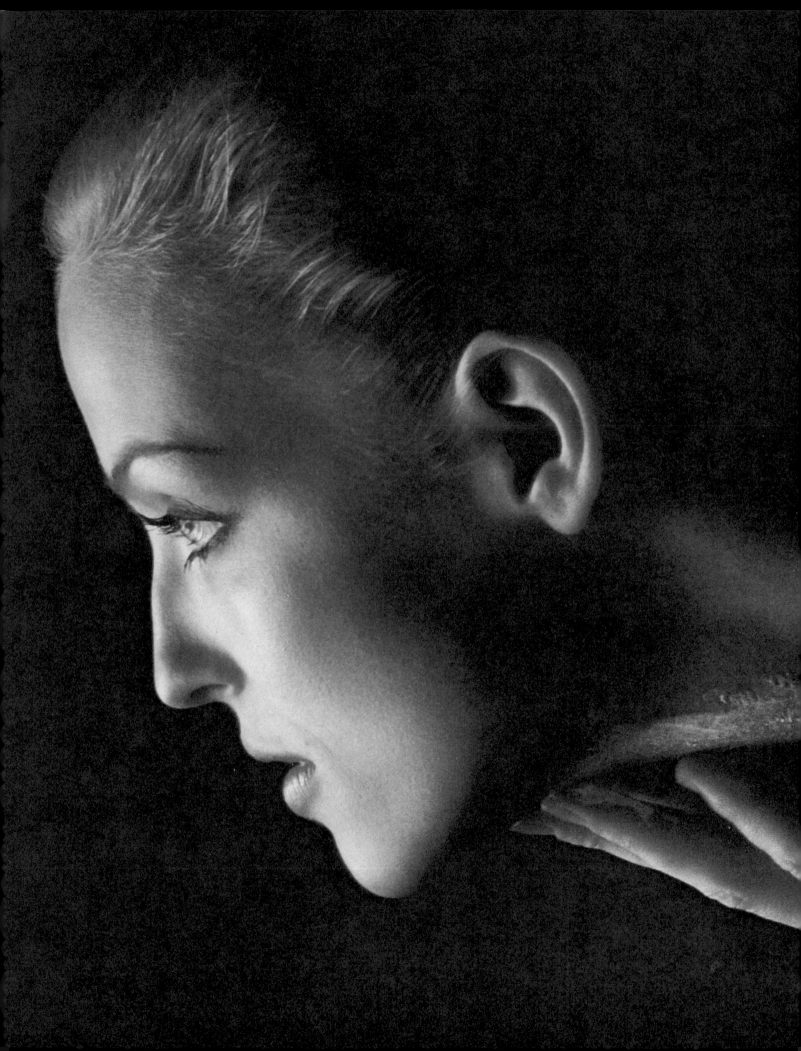

Face and Neck

Your skin is your body's dress. It may be like silk or rough muslin, wrinkle-free or slightly wrinkled. It depends on you. This chapter will tell you how to have a beautiful, well-groomed neck and a silky complexion with few lines. The program outlined here requires you to be conscientious, but the results are worth the time and effort.

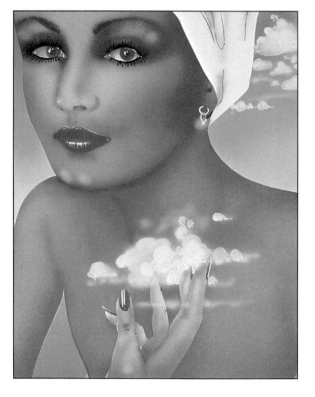

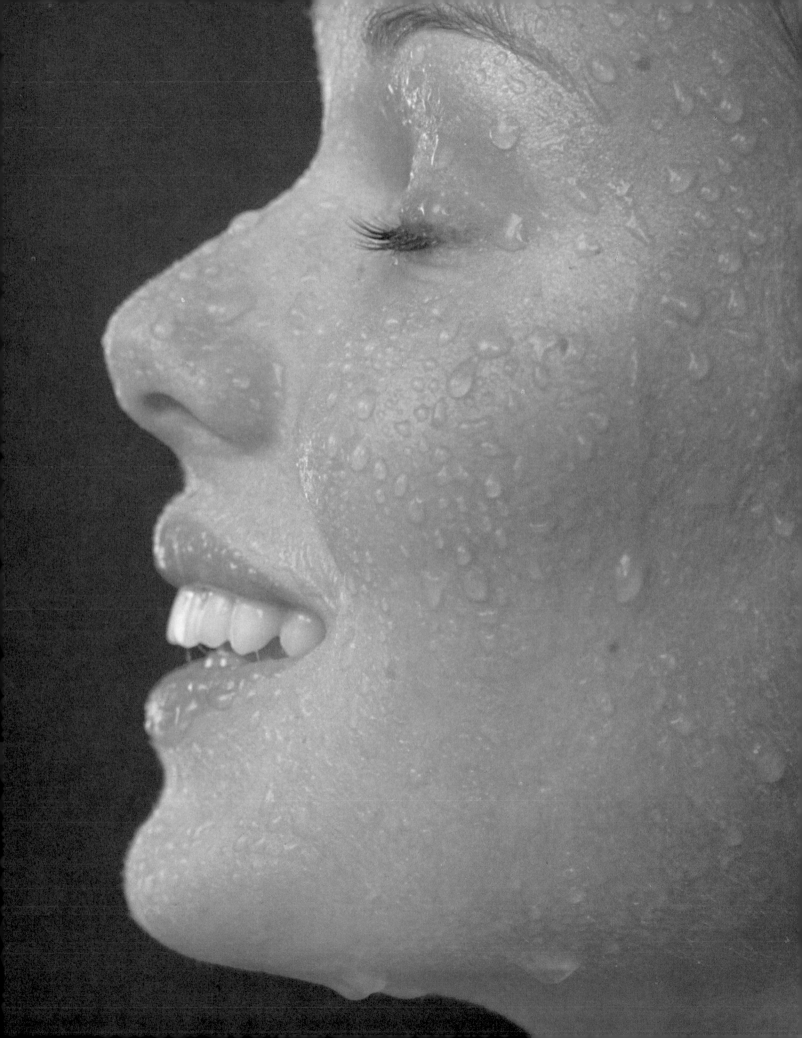

Different Skin Types

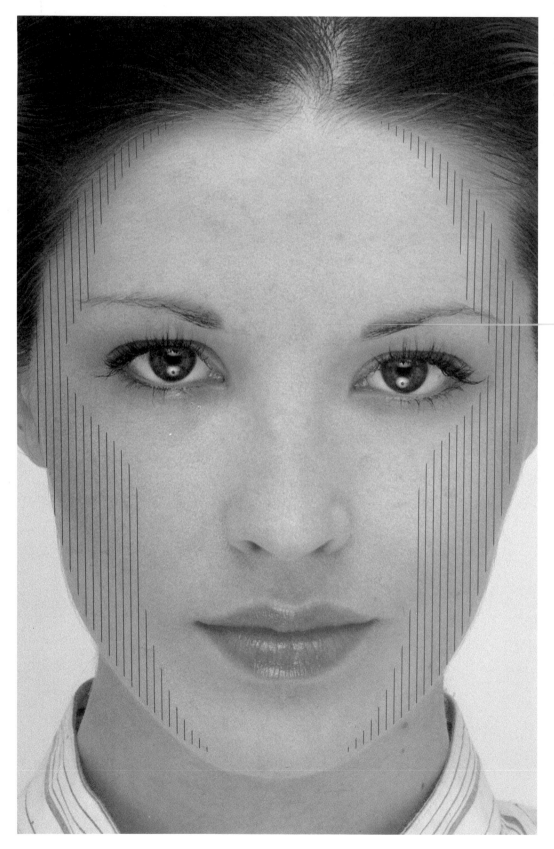

A good skin-care program starts with knowing what skin type you have. A simple test will tell you whether you have normal, dry, sensitive, oily or combination skin.

Wash your face in the evening with soap and water. Don't use moisturizing cream afterward. The next morning, look at your skin in a mirror. Touch your face lightly with freshly washed fingers. You will discover which parts of your face are dry and which parts are oily.

Normal skin will have a very slight layer of oil over the entire surface of the face. This skin type is the easiest to care for and has no major problems. Other skin types have advantages and disadvantages.

Dry skin is thin and delicate, with fine pores. It feels tight after being washed with normal soap. It has a tendency to flake slightly, and develops wrinkles easily. It is not prone to blemishes.

Sensitive skin has most of the characteristics of dry skin. But it itches, burns and becomes inflamed or blemished when exposed to the elements. It also has a tendency to develop allergies to cosmetics and other skin-care products.

Dry skin is susceptible to irritation and wrinkles easily.

Oily skin has large pores. It becomes shiny shortly after being washed. It does not wrinkle easily, but frequently develops blemishes.

Combination skin has both dry and oily characteristics. Usually the forehead, nose and chin are oily and the cheeks, temples and upper lip are dry.

If your skin is dull, rough and susceptible to blackheads, you have dry-oily skin. This condition occurs when underlying layers of skin absorb too much oil. This robs the surface layer of oil it needs to protect itself from cold, wind and sun.

Small blemishes on your face can be caused by illness, stress, lack of proper nutrition or poor hygiene.

You can correct this problem with good skin care and proper eating habits.

Acne is different. If your face is constantly covered with blemishes, you need to consult a dermatologist. Adolescent acne occurs during the hormone fluctuations of puberty. It usually clears up by itself when hormone levels stabilize. However, severe scarring can occur with acne at any age, so a physician's care is always recommended.

Remember that your skin type can change as you age. Be sure to adjust your skin-care program accordingly.

Oily skin can develop blemishes and clogged pores.

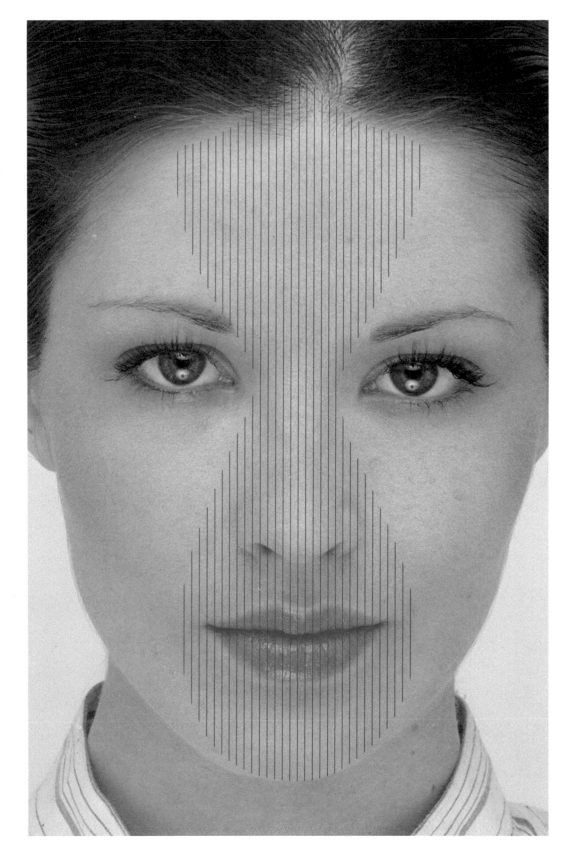

Facial Cleansing

Proper cleansing is the foundation of good skin care. Removing makeup is especially important. If you don't do this every day, your skin will have problems. Oily skin will become more clogged and will develop more blackheads and pimples. Dry skin will become irritated.

If you don't use makeup, you should rinse your face each morning with lukewarm water or a mild astringent. You should wash your face thoroughly each evening.

The major question is, what should you use to wash your face? Dozens of products are on the market, including soaps, oils and creams. The important thing to remember is that the product you choose must match your skin type.

Cleansing Bars containing no perfume are good for young, strong, rather oily skin. This will wash away dirt and natural oil. However, it doesn't remove makeup very well. You need to use a makeup remover for that job.

Your skin type will determine which cleansing product you use.

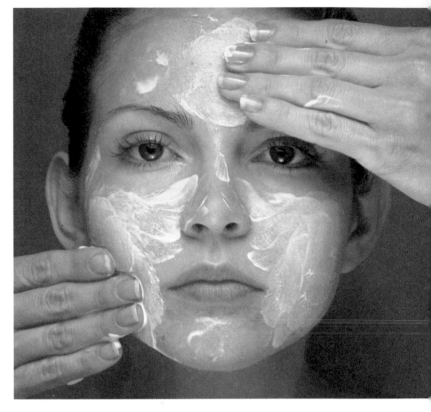

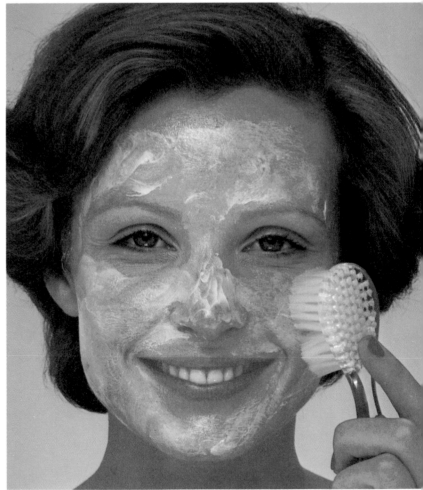

44

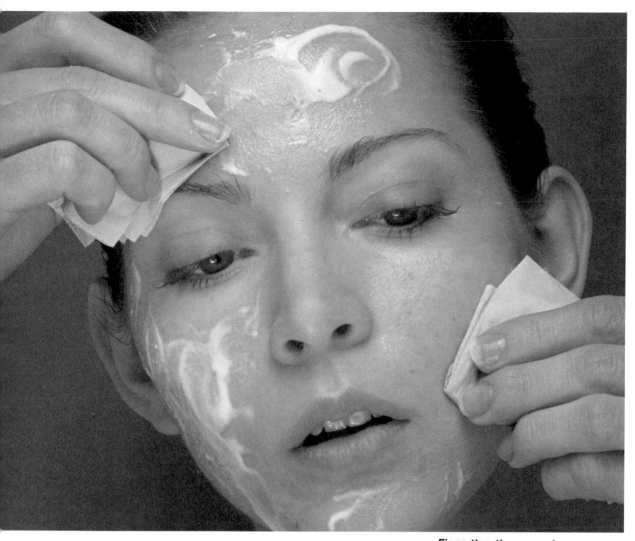

Fingertips, tissues and a soft brush are the tools you'll need for facial cleansing.

Cleansing Lotion is gentle and works well on any type of skin. It removes makeup as well as oil and dirt. Don't use cleansing lotion sparingly. Put plenty of it in the palm of your hand, then massage it into your face with your fingertips.

If the cleansing lotion doesn't contain much oil, you can wash it off with water. Try rinsing your face. If your skin feels sticky, it means the cleansing lotion has a great deal of oil, and you'll have to remove it with dry tissues. Don't try to remove cleansing lotion with cotton balls. They'll leave tiny pieces of lint on your face.

Cleansing Cream works like cleansing lotion, but contains more oil. It is especially good for extremely dry skin.

Use cleansing cream to remove very oily makeup. Apply plenty of cream, then massage it into your skin. Remove it with dry tissues.

Cleansing Oil works like cleansing cream. It works well on normal and oily skin. It is particularly effective for removing oily makeup.

Some cleansing oils are water soluble. You can just rinse them off. Others have to be removed with tissues.

Astringents work in conjunction with cleansing products. They remove excess cleansers and any oil that remains on the skin.

45

Exfoliation (Skin Scrubbing)

Skin that has large pores, blemishes or poor circulation needs special treatment. A massage with a mildly abrasive cream is the best way to make skin smooth and translucent. The technical term for this procedure is *exfoliation*. You will need an exfoliant cream or facial scrub.

Apply an astringent after using a facial scrub. It soothes and relaxes skin.

These products contain oils and cleansing substances which dissolve dirt that doesn't come off with normal washing. They also remove dead skin. Your complexion seems rosier and smoother after such intensive cleansing. But exfoliant creams are only *extra* cleansers. They don't replace daily washing.

With normal to oily skin, you can use these creams once or twice a week. With sensitive skin, you should use them only every 8 to 14 days.

Wash your face the usual way. Wet skin thoroughly, then apply the exfoliant cream. Don't put any around your eyes. Rub the cream in lightly. If you massage too vigorously, you can irritate your skin.

Rinse your face afterward with lukewarm water and carefully apply moisturizer.

After exfoliation, skin will absorb oil and moisture more readily. If your skin has large pores, be sure to use special astringents formulated for this problem.

If your skin is blemished, you don't necessarily have acne. Everyone gets small pimples or blackheads occasionally. You can usually eliminate them by washing your face carefully and watching your diet.

You can remove small pimples and blackheads, but you must do it carefully.

For best results, steam your face, then apply warm compresses. This makes the skin swell slightly.

Wrap a tissue around the first finger of each hand and dip the tissue in rubbing alcohol.

Facial scrubs can be used not only on your face, but also on your chest, back and arms.

Pull the skin around the blackhead apart slightly, then press against the blackhead. Don't press too hard. If the blackhead doesn't come out immediately, leave it alone. If you continue to work on it, it will irritate the skin. This can lead to inflammation, pimples and scars.

Never try to remove a red, inflamed pimple. Disinfect the area with astringent containing alcohol or with antiseptic lotion.

If blackheads or pimples persist or spread, see a dermatologist.

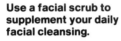

Use a facial scrub to supplement your daily facial cleansing.

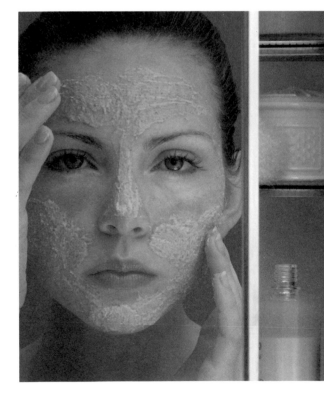

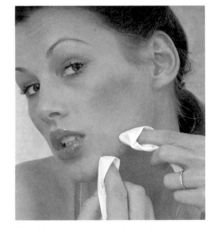

Careful cleansing and good eating habits can help clear up blemishes.

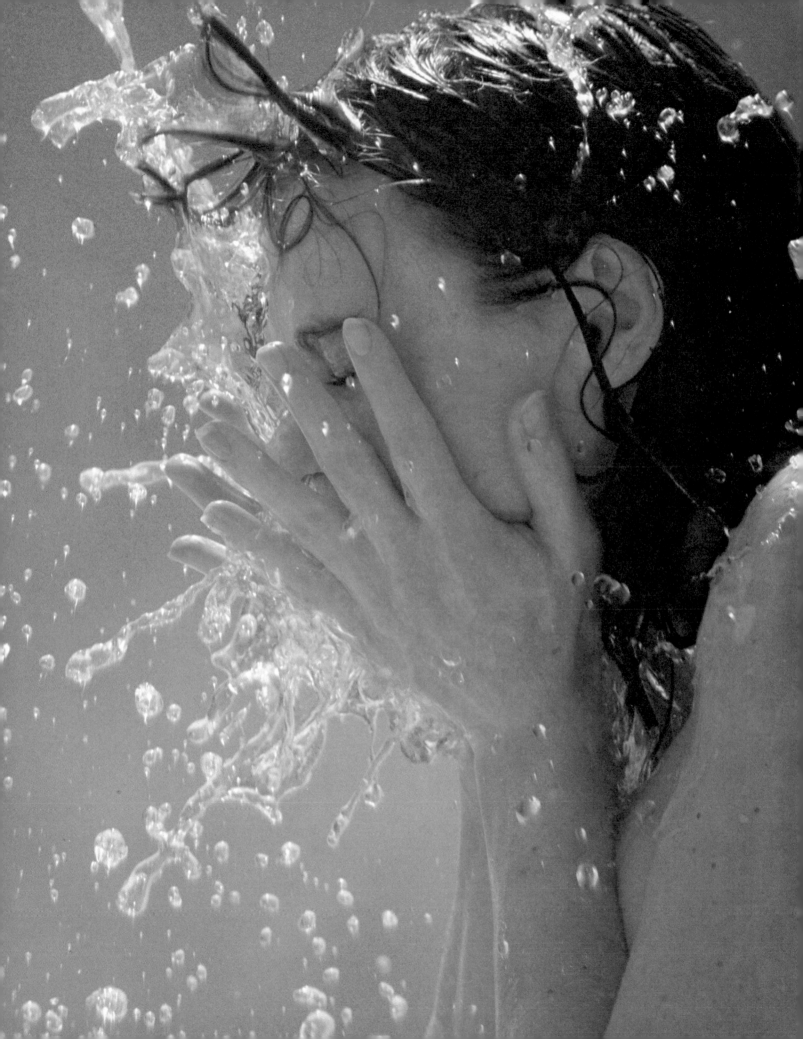

Steaming Your Face

Steaming your face occasionally may be beneficial. It can open the pores, which makes blackheads and pimples easier to remove. It can stimulate circulation, and help facial masks and creams work more effectively.

Try steaming your face every week or two if you have oily or blemished skin.

Steam your face no more than once a month if you have dry skin. Be sure to apply a good moisturizer before you begin your steam treatment.

It is important not to steam your face too often. Frequent steaming might damage your skin.

To steam your face, wash it thoroughly, then pin up your hair. Boil 1 quart of water (4 cups). Put a handful of herbs in a bowl and pour the boiling water over them. Chamomile, sage, peppermint, eucalyptus and lavender disinfect and soothe skin. They also contain oils that are beneficial to sinus passages.

You can also use herbal oils from health food stores. Add 5 or 6 drops for every quart of water.

Bend over the bowl. Drape a large towel over your head so no steam escapes.

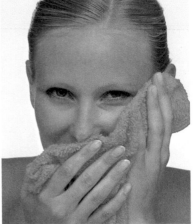

Don't steam more than 10 minutes. When you're finished, dab your face lightly with a soft cloth.

If you need to remove blackheads, wash your skin afterward with the water remaining in the bowl. This will disinfect your skin and help prevent inflammation. Then rinse your face with cool water to close pores.

You can use a warm compress instead of steam. Prepare your boiling water the same way. You can even use the same herbs.

Soak a towel in the bowl, then wring it out. Be sure it is not too hot. Fold it lengthwise and cover your face from chin to cheeks, leaving your mouth and nose free. Let the compress stay in place 2 minutes.

Lukewarm compresses are good for dry and wrinkled skin.

Alternating warm and cold compresses is especially refreshing. Put two bowls next to you. The bowl on the left should contain a warm herbal solution, the bowl on the right a cold one. Put a towel in the warm solution, wring it out and place it on your face for 1 minute. Soak another towel in the cool solution and apply it to your face for 20 seconds. Repeat 3 to 4 times. The last compress should be a cool one.

Vaporized-steam treatments, offered by some beauty salons, have similar effects. Vaporized steam is helpful if you have numerous pimples and blackheads to remove. It also keeps exfoliant creams and facial masks moist while they are on your skin, making them more effective.

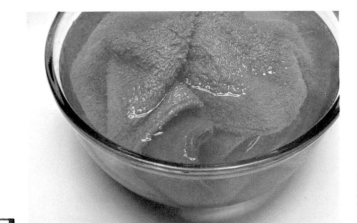

Steaming your face and using compresses will soften rough skin and improve circulation. Adding herbs to the water will help soothe skin.

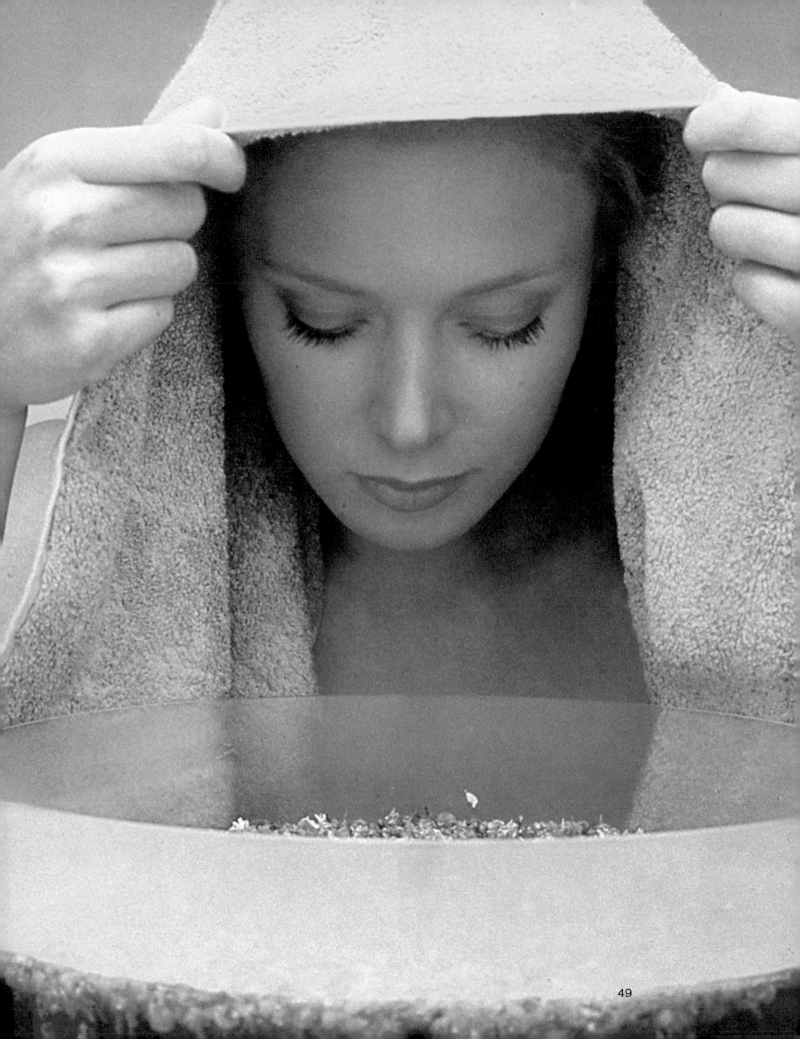

Facial Masks

Masks are quick beauty treatments that also alleviate numerous skin problems. They clean, soothe, tighten and refresh your face while stimulating circulation.

Peel-Off and Cleansing Masks—Peel-off masks and cleansing masks are good for neglected skin or skin with poor circulation.

Peel-off masks are applied either by hand or with a brush. They build up a translucent film on the skin. After a few minutes you can either wash or peel them off. These masks contain mild exfoliants, which give your face a thorough cleansing and gentle massage.

Cleansing masks are applied by hand. They are like a thick cream at first. Then they dry into a hard crust. You wash them off with a towel soaked in lukewarm water. Apply moisturizer afterward.

Cleansing masks stimulate circulation, making your complexion rosier.

Moisture Masks—These creams and gels are very easy to use. You put them on, leave them several minutes, then wipe them off with tissues or a soft, dry cloth. Apply makeup immediately.

Cream masks contain waxes and oils that enable your skin to retain more moisture. They make wrinkles less noticeable for several hours, and give your face and neck a fresh, full look.

Gel masks have ingredients that cool your skin and improve circulation. They make your complexion smooth and pink.

Masks for Blemished Skin—These masks can't cure acne. But they can disinfect and soothe skin, and improve circulation.

Masks for blemished skin can alleviate pimples, but only if you apply them 2 to 3 times a week. They can't eliminate blackheads. You should carefully remove those blemishes before applying these masks.

After you apply the mask, lie down while it dries. Then slowly soften it and remove it with a moist towel and lukewarm water. Afterward, apply moisturizer formulated for oily or blemished skin.

Remember to choose the mask that works best for your skin type.

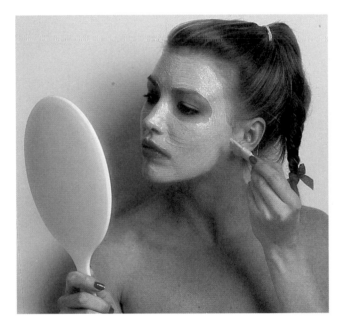

A peel-off mask loosens dead skin and opens clogged pores. Apply this mask with a small brush.

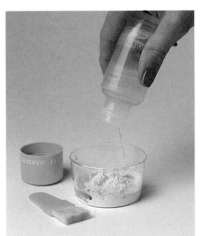

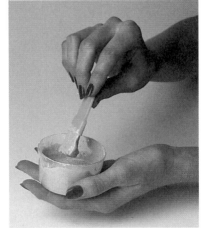

Most masks work well with normal skin. Peel-off masks are especially refreshing.

Dry and sensitive skin react well to moisture masks. The oil and soothing substances in these masks make skin more resistant to irritation.

Relax while your mask is working.

Oily or blemished skin needs peel-off, cleansing or clay masks. These masks remove excess oil from skin and stimulate circulation. They make complexions smoother and prettier.

You must clean your skin thoroughly before applying any mask. Cover your entire neck and face, except lips, nostrils and the skin around your eyes. The eye area should be treated with a moisturizing cream before any mask is applied.

If you are using a peel-off, cleansing or clay mask, apply moisturizer afterward. If you like, you can apply makeup immediately.

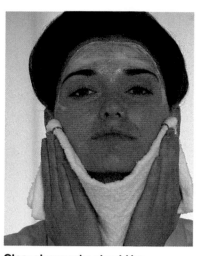

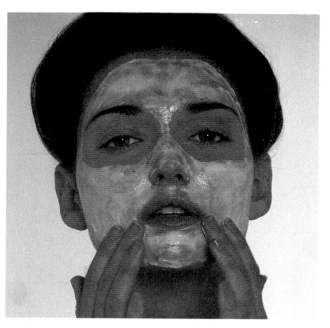

Cleansing masks should be removed with a wet towel. Masks can have a gentle, massaging effect.

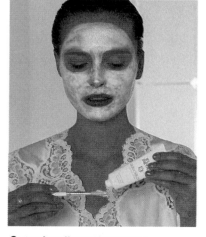

Occasionally apply a mask instead of night cream. Peel-off masks are easy to remove.

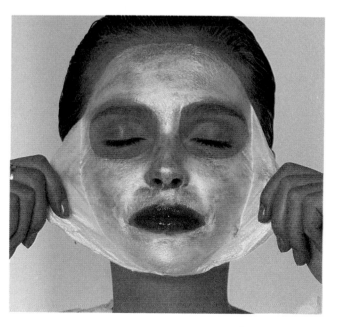

Day Creams and Night Creams

You are never too young or too old to start a skin-care program. Skin is assaulted by wind, sun, hard water, pollutants, chemicals and stress. Day creams enable your skin to withstand these attacks.

Up to age 20, you need to use only a light moisturizer morning and evening. But after that, you need two different creams, one for day and one for night.

Day Creams—Day creams keep the skin's natural moisture from evaporating and supply additional moisturizers. They also act as a makeup base.

Many day creams have sunscreens, which protect the skin from ultraviolet rays. It is especially important that your moisturizer contain a sunscreen if you live in a dry, sunny climate. It can help keep skin from aging as quickly.

A good moisturizer will last all day. If your skin feels tight after 2 to 3 hours, then change products. It's possible that the cream doesn't contain enough moisturizers for your skin.

Even expensive creams can't remove fine lines.

Day creams work best on normal skin or combination skin. If your skin is very dry or sensitive, you need a cream with additional moisturizers. If you have oily skin, ask for an oil-free cream. These preparations work like blotting paper, absorbing excess oil.

If you have blemished skin, use a lightly tinted cream that will cover and disinfect problem areas. Be sure to use a light moisturizer on the rest of your face.

Night Creams—These supply your skin with moisture and oils while you sleep.

They should be more or less oily, depending on your skin type.

Dry or sensitive skin needs a heavy, oily cream. It should provide additional moisturizers and soothe irritation.

Oily or combination skin needs a cream that will clear up small blemishes without removing all oil and moisture. Herbal creams work especially well.

Blemished skin needs a cream that will speed the healing process and prevent inflammation.

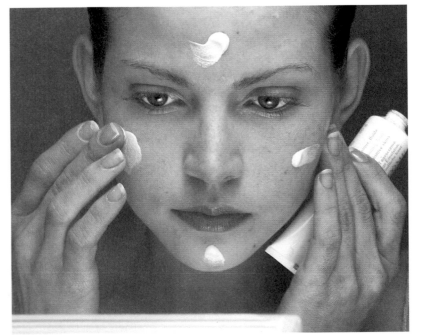

Put several dabs of cream on your face and blend them gently with your fingertips. Always work with circular, upward strokes. Don't rub too vigorously. You'll stretch your skin.

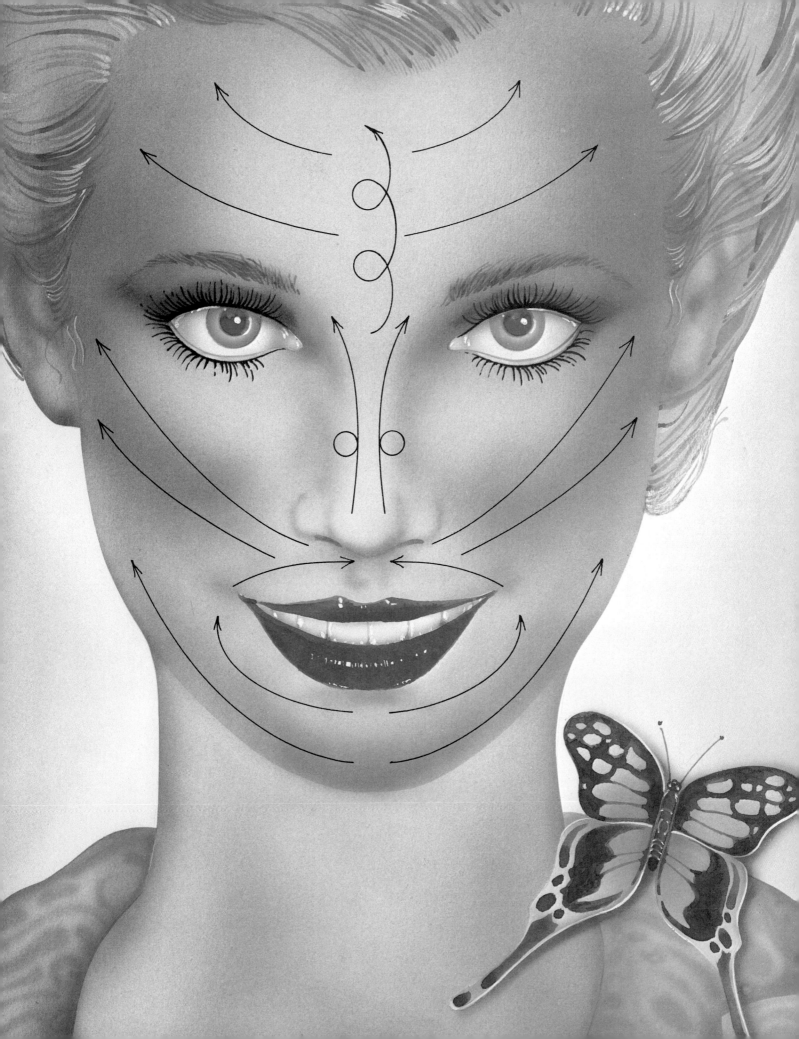

Facial Massage

Your face will be smoother, more youthful and more supple if you have a cosmetologist massage it regularly.

You can also give yourself facial massages. They will be effective only if you do them regularly. You'll get the best results if you massage your face several minutes each day. Try giving yourself massages when you cleanse your face or apply a day or night cream.

Remember that massaging your face incorrectly can harm rather than help your skin. Be sure to follow these four rules:

1. Massage your face very gently, using your fingertips.
2. Don't stretch or pull your skin.
3. Always cleanse your face and apply cream before starting your massage.

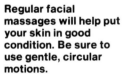

Regular facial massages will help put your skin in good condition. Be sure to use gentle, circular motions.

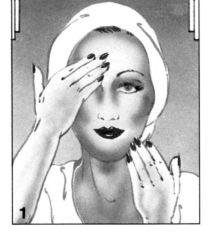

4. Massage your face when you are relaxed and have time to concentrate on the movements. Giving yourself a massage when you're tense and rushed is counterproductive.

You want to concentrate your massage on the parts of the face where the muscles work hardest. These include your forehead, cheeks, mouth, chin, neck, and the areas around your eyes and on the sides of your nose.

You develop tiny lines on these parts of your face because you use them to form your facial expressions. Try to control the types of expressions you use. Your skin will lose its elasticity and develop wrinkles if you constantly frown or raise your eyebrows while talking or thinking. Massages can't

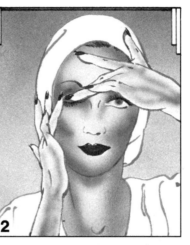

remove wrinkles that already exist.

The illustrations on these facing pages show you how to perform facial massages.

Picture 1

This massage will make your forehead smoother. Put the tips of your first three fingers between your eyebrows, just above your nose. Gently massage toward the brows. Then massage up and across the forehead. Move your left hand toward the left and your right hand toward the right. Repeat 5 times.

Picture 2

These movements are for your eye area. Close your eyes slightly. Put the ring finger of your left hand on the outer corner of your left eye. This finger will hold the skin in place and prevent it from being pulled.

You'll use the ring finger of your other hand to do the massage. Put eye cream on that finger. Starting under your

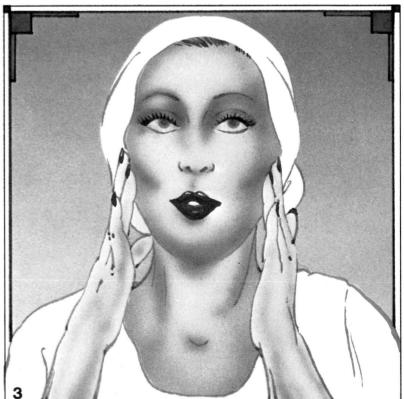

lower lid, move with small, circular motions from the outer corner of the eye to the inner corner. Then go to the upper lid and move from the inner corner to the outer corner. Do this 6 times. Repeat this procedure on your right eyelid. Be sure to massage gently and slowly. The skin around your eyes is very thin and easily damaged.

Picture 3

This helps prevent smile lines. Relax your face, then purse your lips and open your mouth slightly. Put your fingertips beside the lower lip. Massage the skin with light circular motions, moving up and back toward your ears. Repeat 6 times.

Picture 4

This massage will help eliminate a double chin. Sit up straight, bend your upper body slightly forward, then lean your head back. Put your lower lip over your upper lip. This strengthens the neck muscles. Then put the index and second

fingers of your left hand on your chin, and put the two smaller fingers of that hand under your chin. Using small, circular motions, move your fingertips to your ears. Repeat 5 times.

If your neck is developing wrinkles, try this. Lean your head back and toward your right shoulder. Put the fingertips of your left hand flat under your chin. Using small, circular motions, move your fingertips down your neck. Then lean your head back and

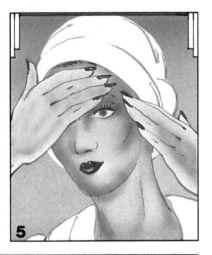

5

toward your left shoulder. Repeat the procedure. Do the entire sequence 5 times.

Picture 5

This massage helps prevent wrinkles on your forehead. Use your left hand to hold your skin in place. Press it just above the right eyebrow. Put the fingertips of your right hand just below your left hand. Rub the side of your head with gentle, circular motions 10 times. Move your left hand an inch to the left. Move your right hand the same distance. Rub this area with circular motions 10 times. Repeat this procedure until you've massaged the entire forehead and temple area.

Picture 6

These movements will help prevent wrinkles between your nose and mouth. Do them

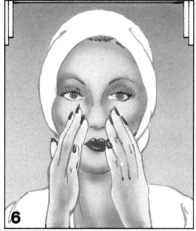

6

Massage these areas of your face to minimize lines:
1. Between your eyes
2. Around your eyes
3. Around your mouth
4. Under your chin
5. On your forehead
6. On both sides of your nose.

quickly while applying cream to your face. Put the index and second fingers of each hand between your eyebrows. Using first the right hand, then the left, move down the sides of your nose with short, circular movements. Then put your fingers at the inner corners of your eyes. Massage down to the corners of your mouth. Repeat 5 times.

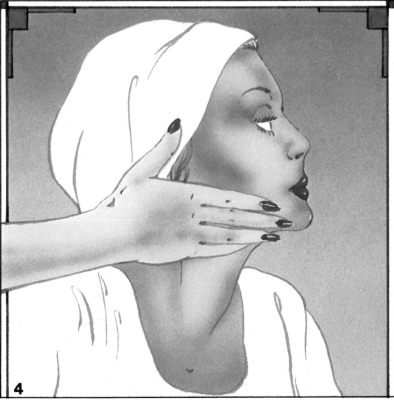

4

Exercises for Your Face

Facial exercises won't work miracles, but they can minimize some existing wrinkles and help prevent new ones.

The photographs on these pages illustrate some very good exercises for your mouth and cheek muscles.

Picture 1
Puff out your cheeks as hard as you can. Then press the air out with your fists. Repeat 10 times.

Picture 2
Purse your lips hard, then relax them. Repeat 10 times.

Picture 3
Pull your mouth first to the right, then to the left. Repeat 10 times. This helps firm chin contours.

Picture 4
Open your eyes as wide as you can, then close them. Repeat 15 times. This helps prevent crow's-feet.

Picture 5
Squeeze your eyes partly closed and wrinkle your nose. Then relax. Repeat 10 times.

This exercise keeps deep lines from developing between your nose and mouth.

Picture 6
Laugh as much as possible. It's good exercise for your mouth.

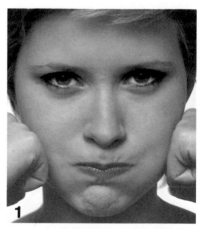

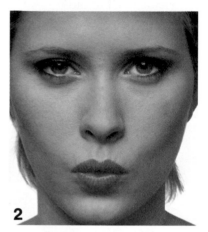

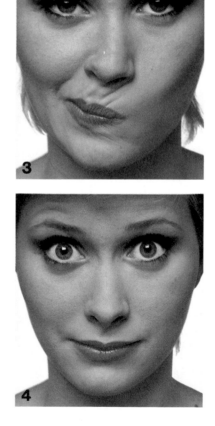

Exercising your face helps prevent wrinkles. So does eliminating bad habits such as wrinkling your forehead and arching your eyebrows.

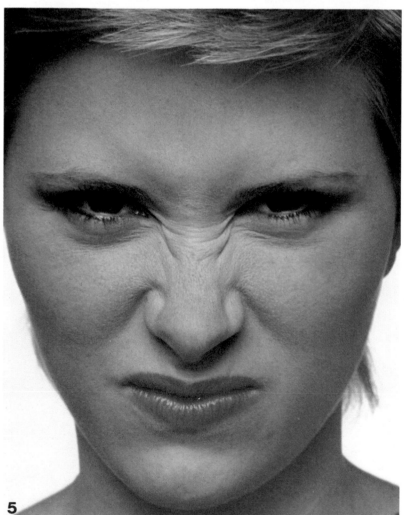

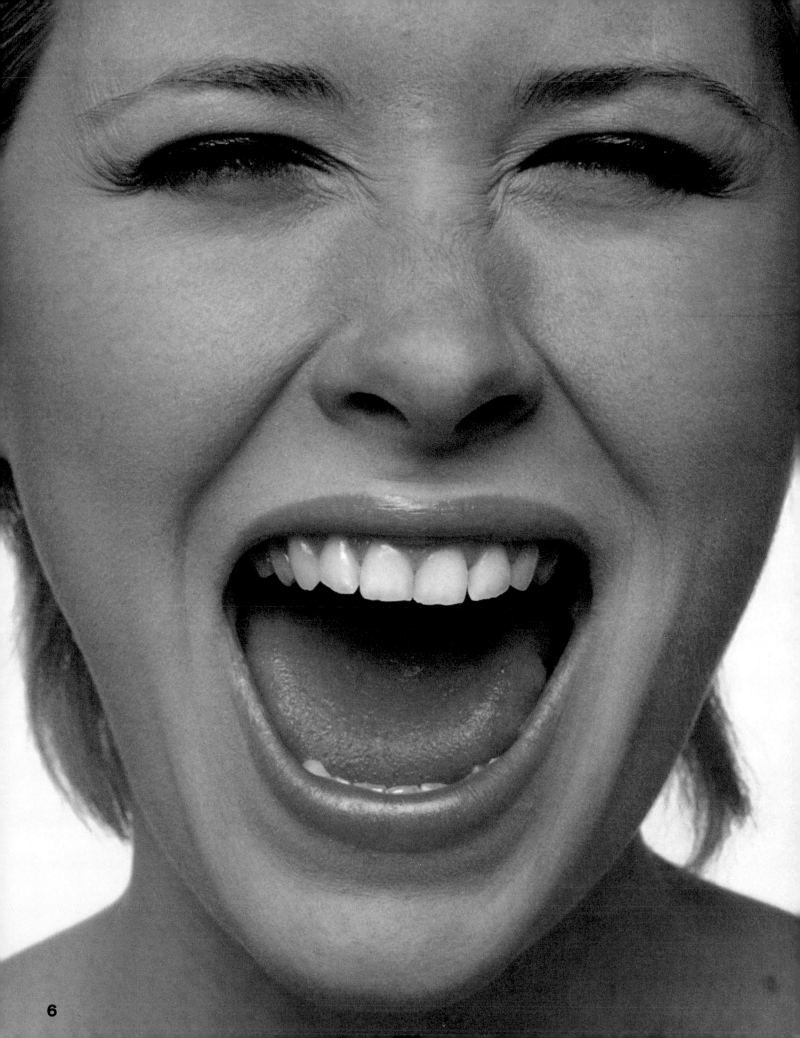

Eye Care

To have beautiful, shining eyes you need more than good makeup. Mascara, eye liner and eye shadow can't make you beautiful if the skin around your eyes is sagging, wrinkled and tired. You have to give the area around your eyes special care. The skin here has fewer sebaceous glands and less supporting tissue.

Because it is so delicate, skin around the eyes tends to become drier and more wrinkled than skin on other parts of your face. Eyelids are also prone to irritation and inflammation.

Proper eye care starts with removing makeup. Don't use your usual skin cleanser to do this in the eye area. It doesn't dissolve mascara, eye liner or eye shadow completely. In addition, some skin cleansers can irritate your eyes.

Dry skin needs special care around the eyes to prevent fine lines.

Eye-makeup remover contains ingredients that dissolve mascara, eye liner and eye shadow completely. They are usually less irritating to your eyes than skin cleansers. Eye-makeup remover is available in oil, cream or lotion form.

Don't use dry cotton balls to apply eye-makeup remover. Lint from these cotton balls can get in your eye. Pads that have been pre-soaked with remover are practical and easy to use.

If you don't have any eye-makeup remover on hand, use baby oil. Put it on a moist cotton ball and move it smoothly over closed lids and lashes.

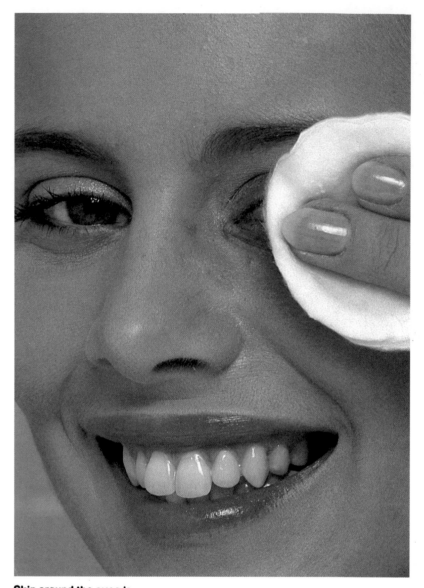

Skin around the eyes is especially sensitive. Be very careful when removing makeup.

Lightly apply eye cream after removing makeup. This special cream moisturizes the skin around the eyes. Don't apply too much and don't get it too close to the edges of the lids.

The cream may get into your eyes during the night and cause swelling and irritation. For best results, dab a little cream around the eye and massage it gently into the skin.

You can also wear eye cream during the day under your makeup.

Cleansing masks and peel-off masks should not be applied in the eye area. Use soft, cream masks or special eye masks instead. They make your skin appear rosier, softer and younger after only 20 minutes. Apply eye masks after cleansing your face, but before using a facial mask. Lie down while the eye masks are working.

Some women have dark circles under their eyes. These occur because the skin in this area is extremely thin. The veins look like shadows. You can minimize these by using a cover stick or concealer. Dab it

If your family has a tendency to develop this condition, it can be alleviated with cosmetic surgery. If the condition results from water retention, other solutions may be available. Water retention can be caused by kidney, circulatory or hormonal problems.

Everyone gets fine lines around their eyes. They are caused by the way we talk, laugh and create facial expressions. How quickly we develop these lines depends on our heredity, lifestyle and beauty program.

If you have dry skin, you'll have a tendency to develop wrinkles at an early age. You'll have to give the skin around your eyes special attention. Be

careful not to pull your skin while applying moisturizers or makeup. If you do, you can stretch your skin, causing it to sag.

You'll also develop lines if you habitually squint. If you're going outside, be sure to wear sunglasses with large, polarized lenses. Frowning, arching your eyebrows and making similar expressions also cause wrinkles.

Fortunately, most of the lines on our face result from smiling and laughing. Don't ever worry about those lines.

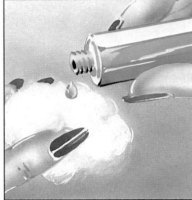

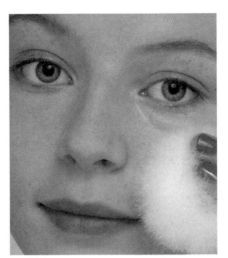

When using cotton balls on your face, make sure no fuzz gets into your eyes.

on lightly, then blend it into your skin with your fingertips.

Some women also develop bags under their eyes. This can be an inherited characteristic. It also can occur when skin and tissue retain too much fat or water.

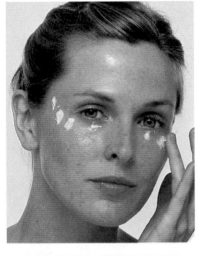

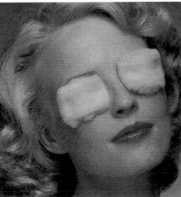

Cream should be dabbed onto sensitive skin and then lightly rubbed in. Compresses will help tired, swollen eyes.

Hints for Tired Eyes

Several remedies can soothe eyes that are tired, burning or swollen. They can sometimes help sagging eyelids, too. These remedies include massage, exercise and compresses.

The illustrations on this page show you how to massage the eye area.

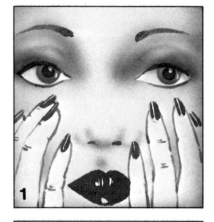

Massage and exercise are good for your eyes, but rest is, too. Close tired eyes for 10 minutes.

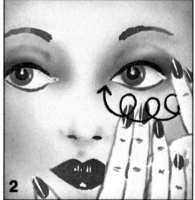

Picture 1
Dab oil or cream on the skin beneath your eye. Don't pull or rub the skin.

Picture 2
Press the index and second fingers of your left hand to the outside corner of your left eye. Move the fingers to the left until the skin has tightened slightly. Massage the skin with the index and second fingers of your right hand. Use gentle, circular motions. Be sure that the skin doesn't wrinkle as you massage it. Repeat the procedure on the area around your right eye.

Picture 3
Put the first three fingers of your left hand on the left side of your head, about 1/2 inch from the outside corner of your left eye. Massage around the eye with the index finger of your right hand. Start underneath the eye at the

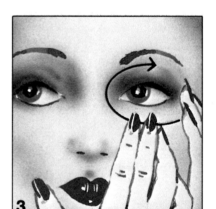

outside corner. Move with light, circular movements to the nose, and then up under the brow.

Picture 4
Close your eyes. Put the index finger of each hand lightly under each eyebrow. Press the second finger lightly against the eyelid. Try to open your eyes against this gentle pressure. Hold for 3 seconds and then relax. Repeat 5 times.

Using creams day and night will help keep your skin soft.

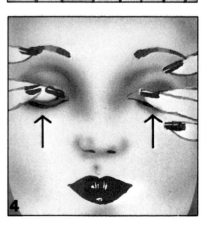

Picture 5
Open your eyes as wide as you can. Press your fingertips against your forehead just above the eyebrows. Use your fingertips to keep the skin beneath the brows from sagging. Hold your eyes open wide for 5 seconds. Then release your fingertips and relax your eyelids. Repeat 5 times.

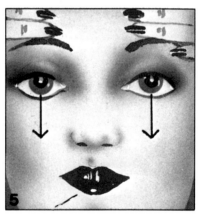

You don't need much time for these eye massages. For best results, do them in the morning. They will relax your eyes and stimulate circulation in the eye area.

Eye exercises relieve eyestrain, which results from studying, reading, writing or watching television. You can minimize eyestrain if you stop your activity for 2 to 3 minutes each hour and focus on something across the room.

The following eye exercises are easy to do and take only moments. Be sure to do them slowly.

Close your eyes but don't squeeze them shut. Roll them to the left, to the right, then in a circle. Repeat 5 times.

Stare for 5 seconds at a large letter in a magazine or a book. Then stare into the distance 5 seconds. Repeat 5 times.

Open and close your eyelids as fast as you can 15 times. Then do this with your left eyelid while keeping the right eye open. Repeat, using your right eyelid and keeping your left eye open.

Eyedrops can soothe your eyes, but only if you don't use the drops too often. Frequent use can irritate your eyes.

The illustrations on this page show additional exercises. Open your eyes as wide as you can. Move them in a circle. Look all the way to the right, then to the left. Focus on the tip of your nose, then look straight up. The pupils have to be in each position for several

seconds. Be sure not to wrinkle your forehead while doing this exercise. Repeat the movements 10 to 15 times.

Remember that rest is also good for your eyes. Simply close them and relax for a minute or two.

Eyedrops can refresh tired eyes, but you shouldn't use them too often. Frequent or long-term use can irritate your eyes, making them look bloodshot. Put drops in your eyes no more than once or twice a day for no more than 3 consecutive days.

Eye compresses can relieve swollen lids. In some cases they can also alleviate bags under your eyes. First, remove your eye makeup. Then boil 2 teabags. Let them cool in the refrigerator. Put them on closed eyelids for 10 minutes.

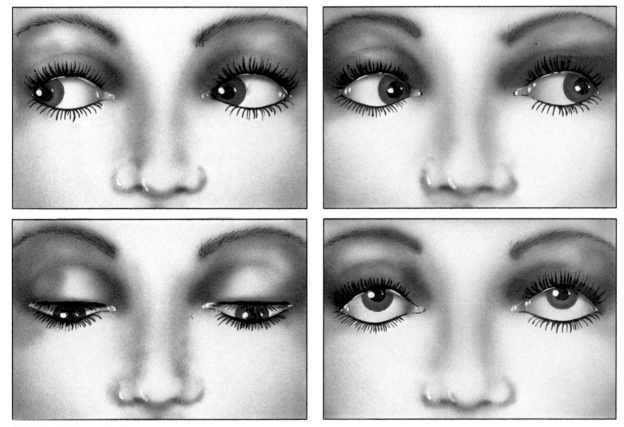

You can wake up tired eyes with exercises.

Neck

Wrinkles usually develop on your neck before they do on your face. This occurs because the skin on the neck is drier and thinner.

If you have sagging skin in this area or a double chin, don't give up. Cosmetics, massage and good posture can minimize these problems.

You must start by treating your neck as carefully as your face. Use a mild cleansing lotion or cream and an alcohol-free astringent in this area.

The most healthful sleeping position for your neck is on your back. Your pillow should be small and hard, so your head will not fall toward your chest.

Oil makes the skin on your neck smooth and supple. Apply plenty of body lotion or moisturizer.

Several exercises will help keep your neck in shape even if you do a lot of desk work. Bend your head back as far as you can. Then forward as far as you can. Repeat 10 times. Bend your head to the right as far as you can, then to the left as far as you can. Repeat 10 times. Circle your head slowly to the right 10 times. Then circle to the left 10 times.

If you have a double chin, try this. Stick out your tongue as far as you can. Try to touch it to the tip of your nose, then to the tip of your chin. Repeat 10 times.

If you have dry skin, you can use your regular facial creams on your neck. These products contain plenty of oil, so your neck will get enough moisturizers.

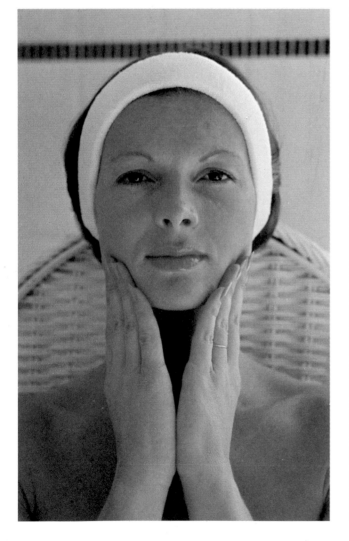

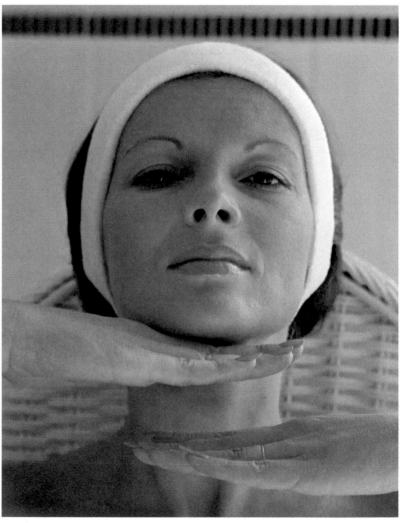

If you have oily or combination skin, you'll need special creams for your neck. Your facial creams will contain little or no oil.

When you apply cream, give your neck a light massage. You can also give your neck a gentle massage while you bathe. If you want to massage with a brush, use the softest you can find. The skin on your neck is very susceptible to damage.

Even the best care won't make your neck pretty if your posture is poor. Think about the position of your head. Hold it erect and look straight ahead. Put your shoulders back. This will help prevent the development of lines and a double chin. It will also make you appear taller and thinner.

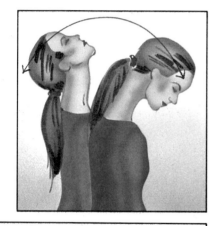

Frequently Asked Questions

Can you create your own facial masks?

Yes. You can't store them, however, so use only the ingredients you need for one mask. Here are three recipes:

For oily skin, pour 1 pint boiling water (2 cups) over 1 heaping teaspoon rosemary and 3 teaspoons sage leaves. Let it steep 15 minutes. Strain the tea and let it cool. Mix tea with facial-mask clay, which is available in beauty supply stores.

For dry skin, mix 1/2 avocado, 1 egg yolk and the juice of 1/2 lemon.

You can also use yogurt as a refreshing moisture mask. Simply put it on your face and leave it 15 minutes. Then gently wash it off.

Is it possible to prevent red, splotchy veins?

It depends. These veins can be caused by numerous factors, including exposure to the sun, topical steroids, liver disease, connective tissue disease and pregnancy. Certain groups of people, including those with fair skin or of Celtic origin, have a tendency to develop these veins more easily than other groups. This tendency can also run in families.

If these veins are an inherited characteristic, there is not much you can do. However, anyone concerned

about this condition should follow certain basic rules. Don't use any creams that make your skin too warm or too cool. Don't use masks that stimulate circulation. Don't use astringents with a high alcohol content. Avoid anything that irritates your skin. Stay out of cold air and wind as much as possible.

You shouldn't sunbathe at all. The heat can enlarge your veins, making them more visible. If you do sit in the sun, use a sunblock.

Saunas and long, hot baths are not good for your skin if you have unsightly red veins. Neither is steaming your face.

If you have this condition, consult a dermatologist. Superficial cautery of these veins may alleviate the condition.

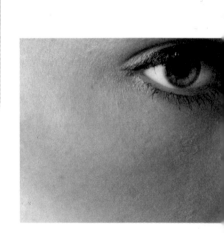

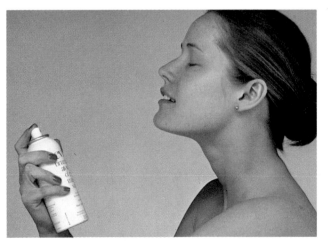

If you have irritated or inflamed skin, don't use any products that stimulate circulation. These include astringents and rubbing alcohol.

Should you always use the same skin products?

No. Your skin changes with age, the seasons, and the places you live and visit. Pregnancy, stress and diet also affect your skin. You should use the products that are best suited for your skin type at the moment.

You can also develop allergies to products that you have used for years. If you change products, you usually can eliminate irritation and swelling.

Does your physical condition affect your looks?

Yes. And it does so to a greater extent than we used to think. For example, research has shown that skin is substantially affected by hormones. Your hormone balance is dependent to a great extent upon your physical condition. If you are under a lot of stress, the levels of some hormones can be affected.

Does soap affect the acid layer on the surface of the skin?

Yes. This layer is a thin film of sweat and oil that covers the surface of the body. It keeps the body from losing too much moisture and prevents bacteria from penetrating the skin. This layer is called *acid* because its chemical reactions are like those of other acidic substances. Soap, on the other hand, is alkaline. When you use soap, you strip some of the acid layer off the skin. Detergent soaps, such as deodorant soaps, are quite harsh and can irritate skin. Try using cleansing bars instead, especially those containing oils. These bars look just like soap, but are milder. Make sure the package says, "acid-balanced" or "pH-balanced."

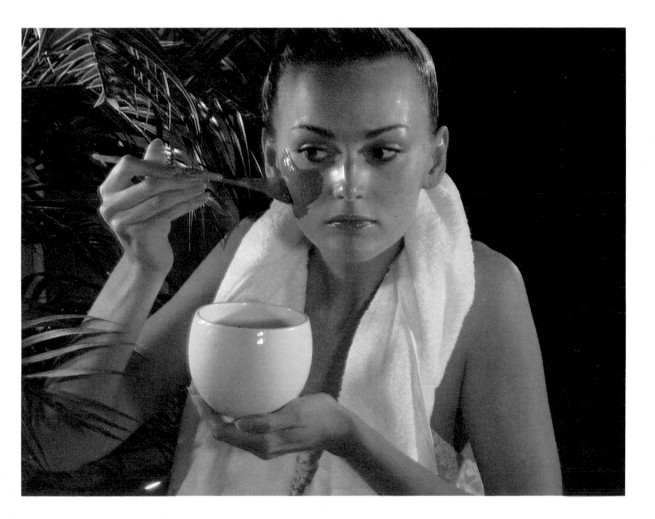

Frequently Asked Questions

Are additives in cosmetics harmful?

Not in small amounts. Additives can sometimes cause allergic reactions. But cosmetics with small amounts of additives are potentially less harmful than cosmetics that have none. For example, products that have no preservatives can become contaminated with bacteria or mildew after one use. The same is true of homemade products. People with sensitive skin can use hypoallergenic products, which don't have the types of additives that usually irritate skin.

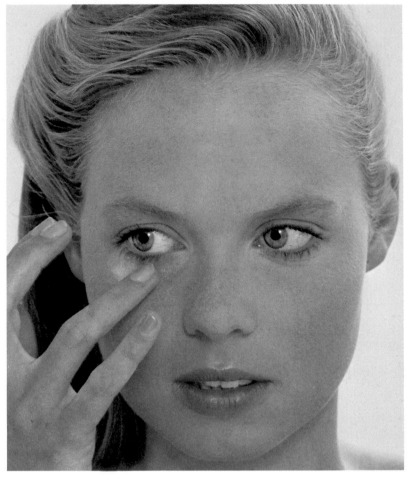

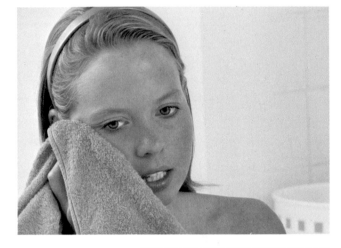

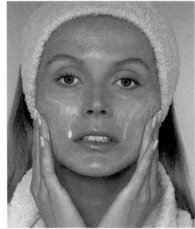

Is it harmful to use makeup without applying a day cream on your skin first?

No. You will not damage your skin if you put makeup directly on it. The pigments in makeup will not penetrate the skin's surface. Even so, there are good reasons for applying day cream underneath makeup. Cream has moisturizers and other substances that protect the skin. Makeup does not. In addition, cream acts as a buffer between your skin and your makeup. This keeps makeup looking fresher longer. Makeup becomes moist and changes color when it comes into contact with the natural oils and perspiration on your skin.

Can stress damage your looks?

Yes. Tension, excitement and worry etch themselves on your skin. It becomes drawn, pale and prone to blemishes. It may also become oilier or drier than normal. Stress also leads to sleeplessness and indigestion, which in turn aggravate skin problems.

Even healthy skin can develop spots and blemishes if you're under stress. They'll disappear once you relax and give your skin special treatment.

Is acne related to diet?

This is a very controversial subject. Many doctors do suspect that there is a link between acne and diet. They recommend that people with acne avoid any food that seems to aggravate the condition. They also recommend that acne sufferers experiment with their entire diet until they find the food plan that produces the fewest skin problems. Such diets usually comprise plenty of grains, fresh fruits and vegetables.

Some doctors feel hormones in meat and chicken may also aggravate acne in some people. These hormones get into the food chain when they are fed to animals to fatten them for slaughter.

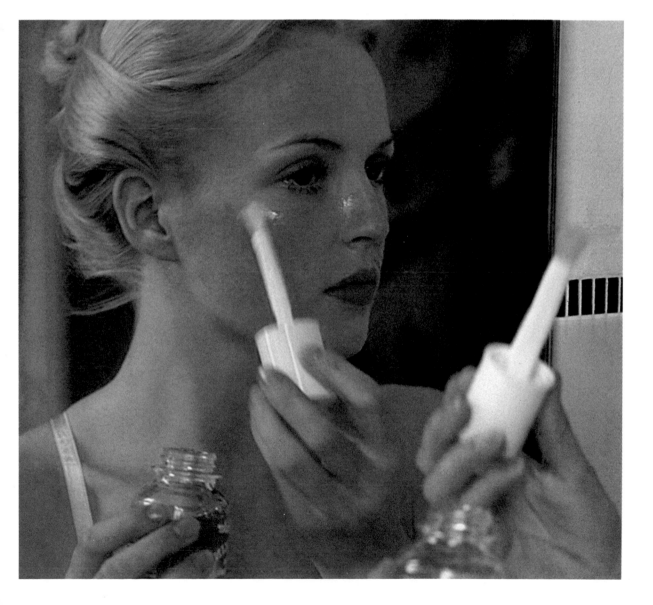

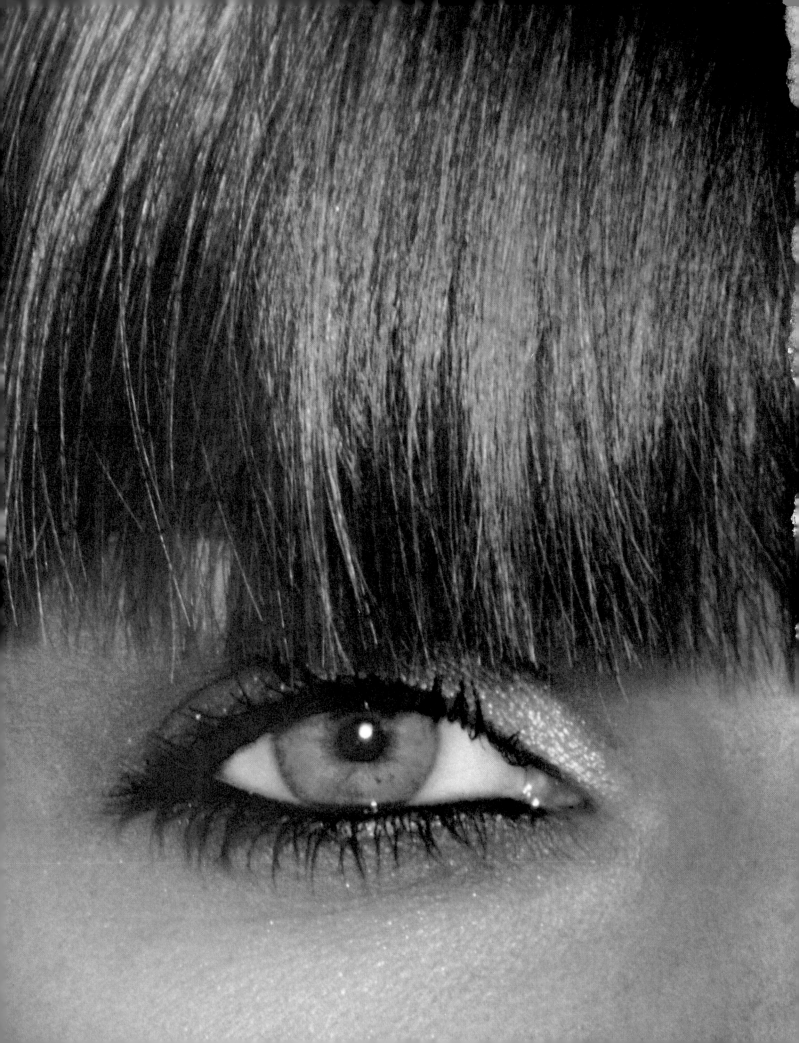

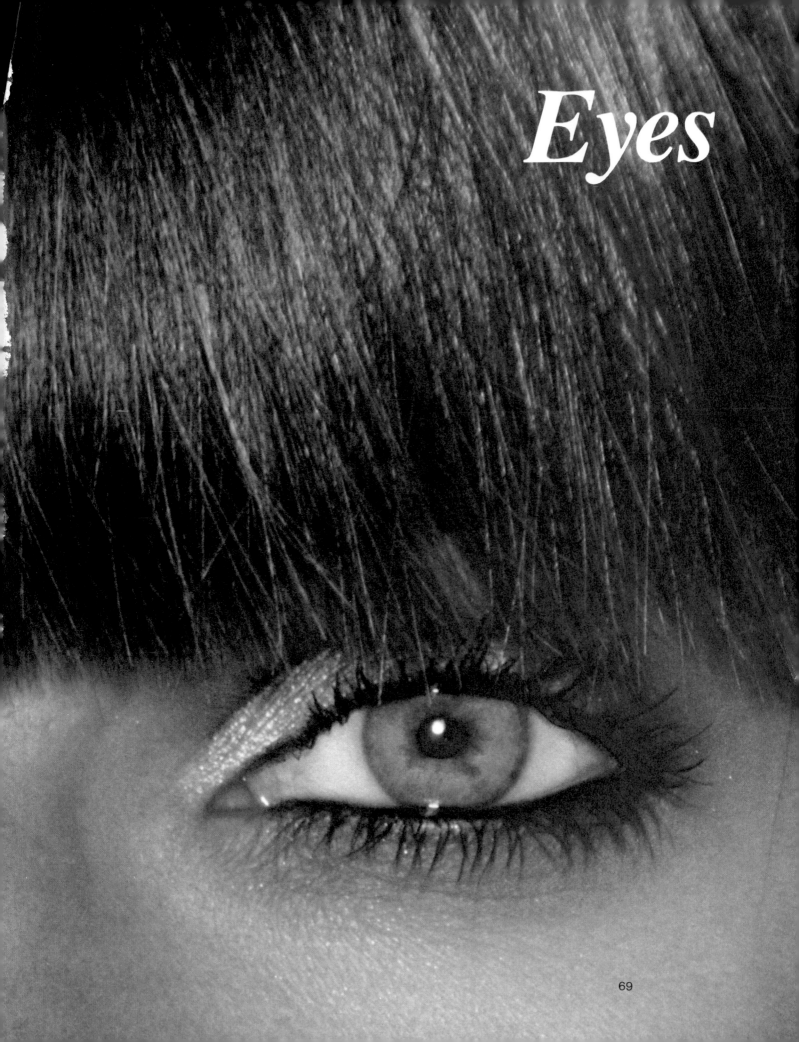

Eyes

When it comes to beauty, the eyes have it. They make the first and most lasting impression on people you meet. They convey your inner self—your personality and your mood. Be sure your eyes tell people what you want them to know at first glance. People will see what you mean if your eyes have thick lashes, nicely shaped brows and perfect makeup. If you have some facial flaws, you can put them out of sight by using the appropriate cosmetics. After all, the hand can sometimes be quicker than the eye.

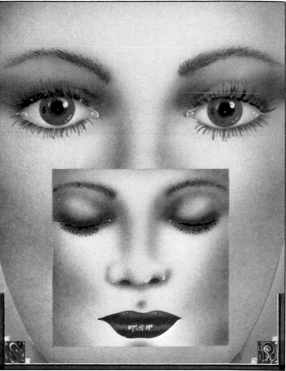

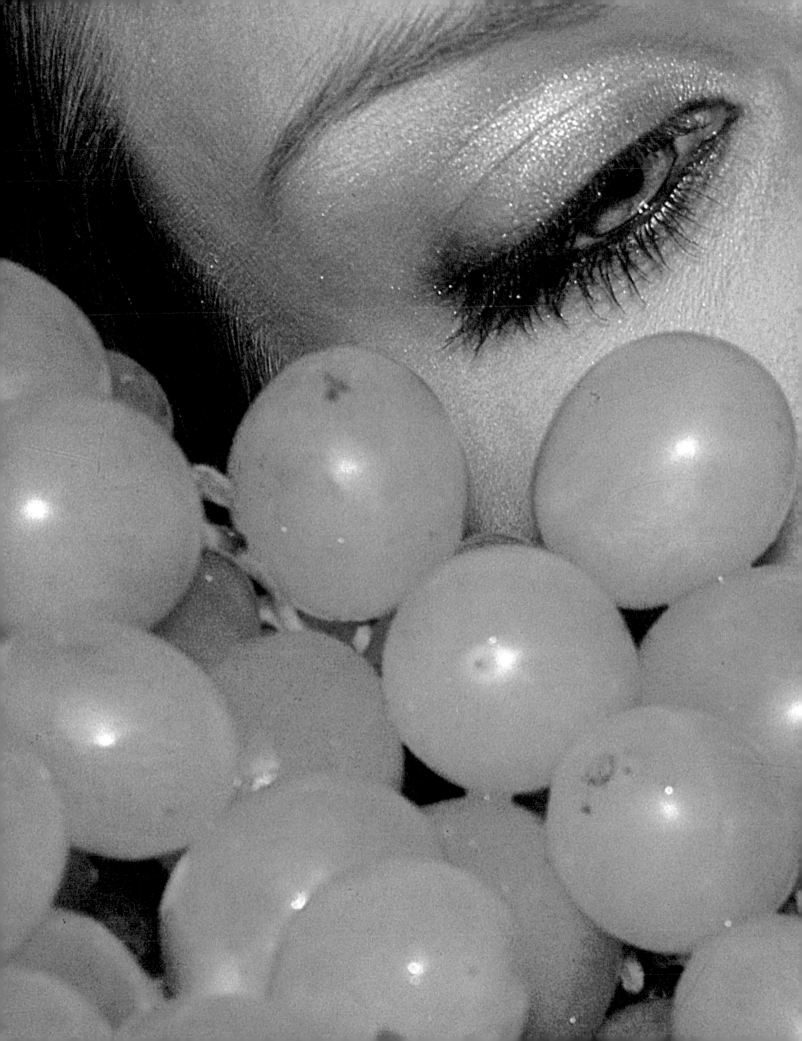

Shaping Your Eyebrows

The shape and color of your eyebrows play a decisive role in forming the overall expression of your face. It is important that the inner edges of the eyebrows begin directly over the inner corners of the eyes. The outer edges should end over the outer corners of the eyes.

You should pluck only the hairs under the brows and between the eyes. Use an astringent with a high alcohol content beforehand.

If you have a square or rectangular face, your eyebrows should be slightly arched. With an oval face, the brows should be straight. If your face is round, your eyebrows should be arched. A heart-shaped face looks prettiest with rounded brows.

Don't paint a thick black line over your brows. Just go over them lightly with an eyebrow pencil. Use a color that matches the natural color of your brows.

After applying eyebrow pencil, brush the brows lightly with an upward motion.

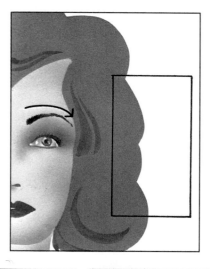
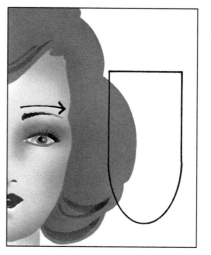
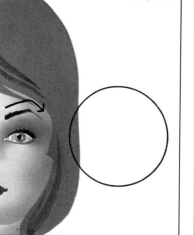
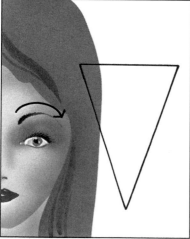

You can shape your eyebrows more effectively if you remove only the hair on the underside of the brow.

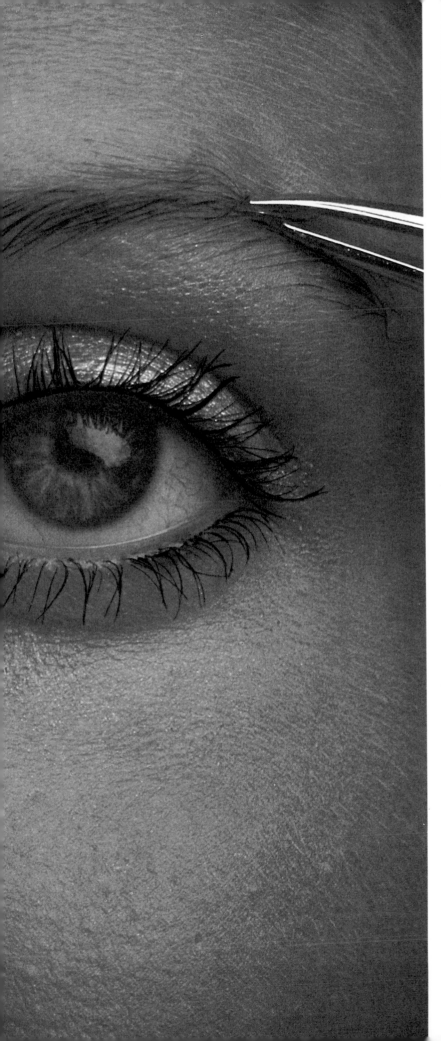
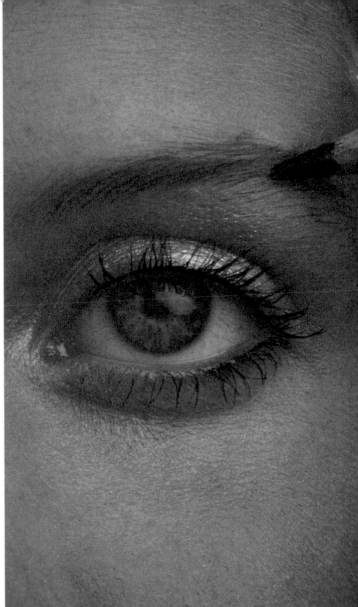
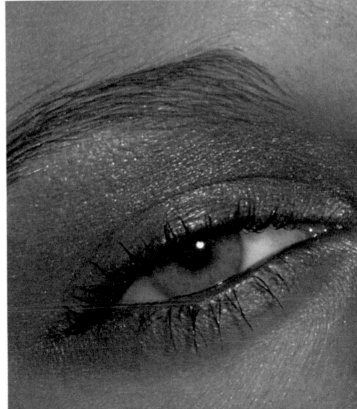

Eye Makeup

Start by putting concealer under your eyes. Apply eye shadow and eye liner. Then curl your lashes and put on mascara.

Eye shadow comes in pencil, cream or powder form. Translucent eye shadow looks prettier and more natural than other types. Eye shadow should accentuate the color and shape of your eyes. It should be discreet in the daytime, and should shine and glitter in the evening.

If you're not sure what color is best for you, try a soft color that matches your eyes and harmonizes with your clothing. It's hard to go wrong if you use light gray, blue, brown or green.

Color sticks are available for eyes, lips and cheeks. They are easy to use and ideal for a quick touch-up.

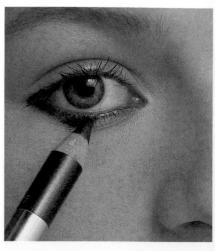

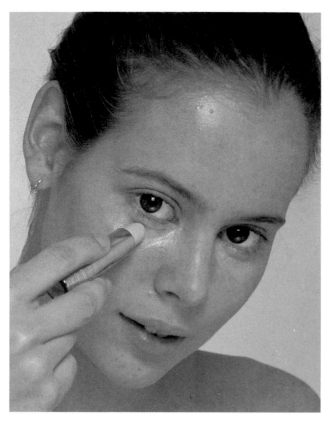

Before you apply foundation, cover dark circles under your eyes with concealer. If you curl your eyelashes, do so before applying mascara.

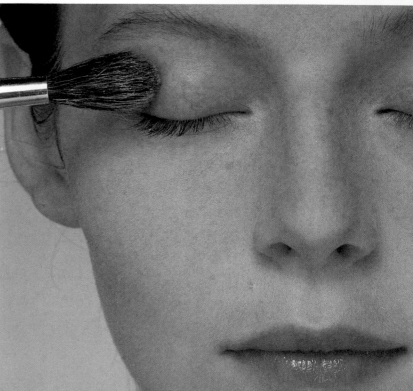

Use pencils directly on your eyelids. Apply creams with your fingertips or a sponge-tipped applicator. Most creams are waterproof, so you can wear them on rainy days or while swimming. Apply powders with applicators.

Apply eye shadow sparingly. If you use pencils, make sure they are soft. They can damage the sensitive skin around your eyes if they are too hard. Hold the pencil over a flame before you put it on your eyelids. This will soften the point and ensure that the color will go on your eyelids smoothly and easily.

With creams, put a little on the back of your hand. Gently rub your fingertips in it, then smooth it on your eyelids.

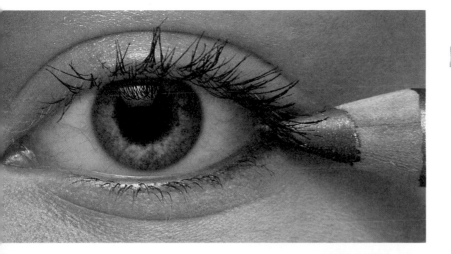

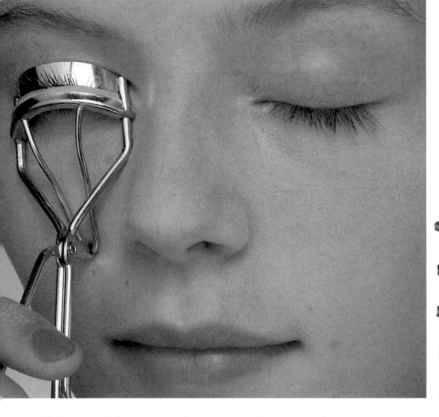

Before applying eye shadow powders, blow the excess off the applicator.

Start applying eye shadow in the middle of your eyelid. Blend it toward the outside corner, then the inside corner. Be sure to blend in the top edge, too.

You can make your eye shadow more dramatic if you put highlighting cream or powder on top of it. These finishing touches must be applied with a light hand, however. Otherwise, your eyelids will look as if they have a glittery white film over them.

Eye-Makeup Techniques

You need a delicate touch when applying eye liner. If your strokes are too heavy, the lines will be too wide or uneven. Before applying eye liner, place a large mirror on a table. When you put the eye liner on, rest your arms on the table.

Make sure that no hair is sticking to the eye-liner applicator. Such hair can easily get into your eyes.

Using the first two fingers of your left hand, pull down the lower eyelid. Gently line the top edge. Close your eyes tightly for several seconds. This will transfer some color to the lower edge of the upper eyelid.

Then make a fine line under the lashes on your lower eyelid. This will make the lashes look thick and pretty. If your lower lashes are thin or sparse, simply touch the eye liner between each lash.

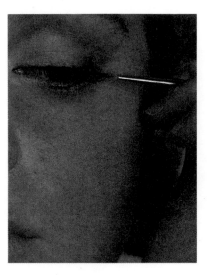

Close your eye and hold down the lashes of the upper lid with the index finger of your left hand. Gently draw a line from the inner corner to the outer corner of your eye.

If you want a more subtle look, line only the outside corner of your upper and lower lids.

You can camouflage beauty flaws in your eye area with some simple tricks. If your eyes are too close together, make your eye shadow and eye liner slightly darker and heavier toward the outside corners of your eyes.

If your eyes are too far apart, make your eye shadow darker toward the inside corners of your eyes. Let the inside edges of your eyebrows extend past the inside corners of your eyes.

Makeup can conceal your eyes' shortcomings.

If your eyes are too small, keep your eyebrows very thin. Use a light eye shadow and highlighting cream or powder. Apply plenty of mascara.

If your eyes are too deep-set, use a very light shadow. Apply a darker shadow on the top of your eyelid. Then put a highlighting cream or powder in the center of the lid.

If your eyes protrude, use a dark eye shadow. Put highlighting cream or powder on the inside and outside corners of the eyelids.

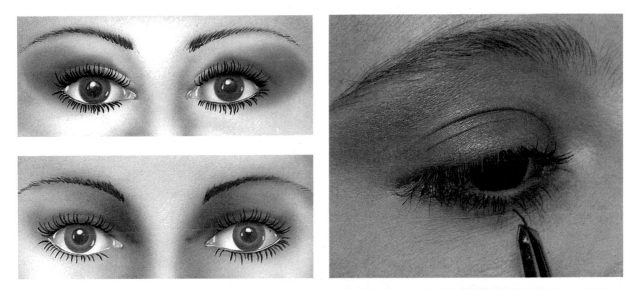

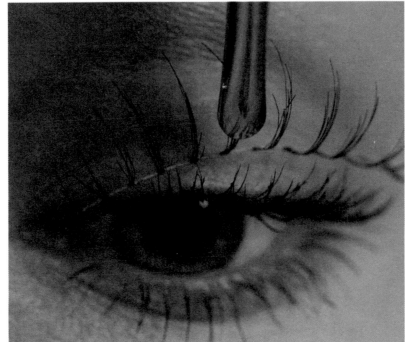

If your own lashes seem too thin, use false ones. Individual lashes, which you apply with tweezers, look more natural than other types. With cosmetics, you can make your eyes seem farther apart or closer together.

Mascara

Mascara will make your lashes look thick and dark. You don't necessarily have to use brown or black mascara. This cosmetic is also available in gray, blue and green. Try several shades until you find the one best suited to your eye color and complexion.

Be sure your eyelashes are clean before you apply mascara. It will form tiny lumps on your lashes otherwise. Curl your lashes before putting on mascara.

If you want your lashes to look natural, you have to apply mascara lightly. Take the applicator and gently brush the lashes on your upper eyelid. Move from the bottom of the lashes to the top. Brush them several times, until every lash has some color. Be sure to get the small, thin lashes in the corner of your eye.

If you have thick, heavy lashes, use a metal applicator. It separates individual lashes more effectively.

You can separate lashes that stick together with a lash brush or lash comb. If you get tiny lumps of mascara on your lashes, gently wipe them off with a tissue or cotton swab.

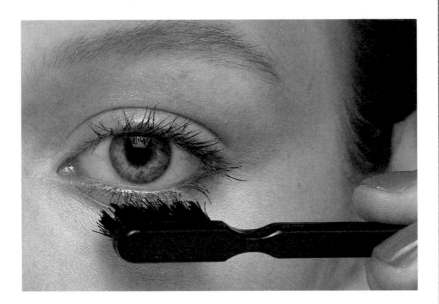

Buy mascara several times a year to ensure that it is fresh and moist when you use it. Mascara crumbles when it dries and becomes difficult to apply. Lashes should be brushed gently afterward.

Apply mascara to the lashes on your lower lid the same way.

You can take off mascara with cold cream or eye-makeup remover. It's important to completely remove all mascara every night. If you don't, your lashes will start to break. This occurs because mascara forms a film over your lashes, making them brittle. The lashes then break when they come in contact with your pillow.

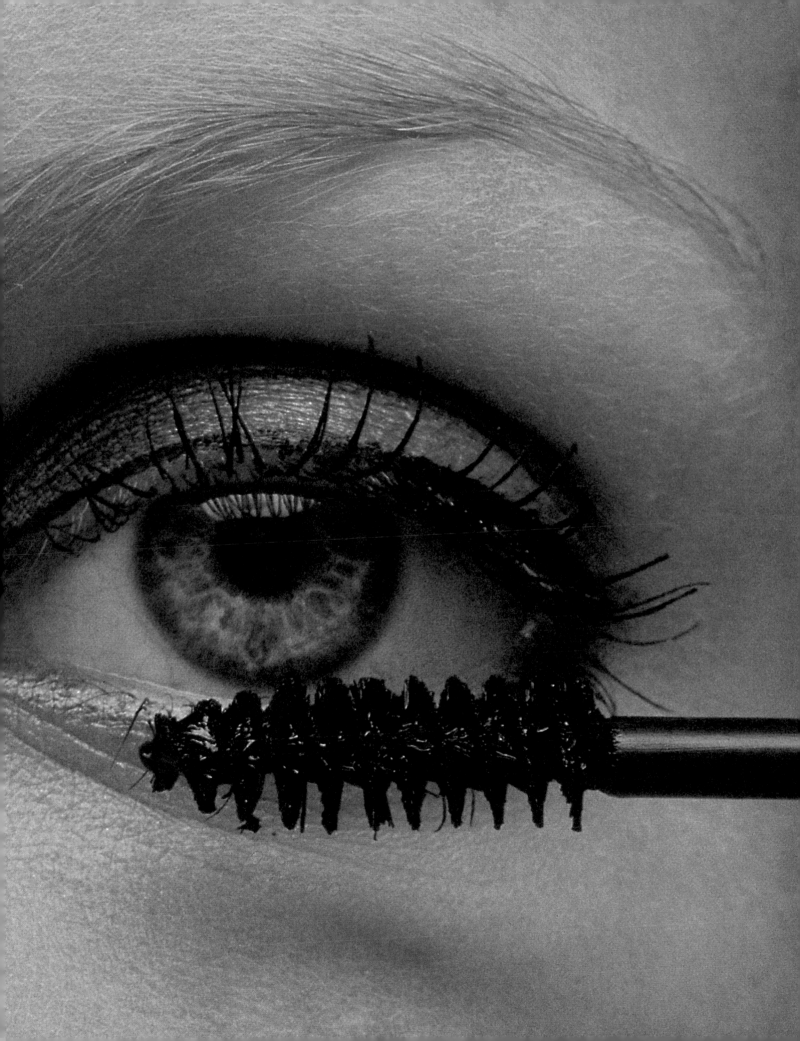

Makeup with Contact Lenses

You have to be careful about applying makeup if you wear contact lenses. Your eyes are very susceptible to irritation.

Usually the eye gets rid of foreign particles by moving the lids or activating the tear ducts. These defense mechanisms don't work as well if you have contact lenses. Particles can get stuck under the lenses. The eye starts to burn and becomes red. Sometimes these particles can also scratch the surface of the eye. This injury is extremely painful and can lead to corneal scarring and diminished vision.

Soft lenses have another major disadvantage. They are very porous and can absorb any makeup that runs into the eye. This can result in irritation and infection. Be sure to sterilize these lenses every night and have them checked regularly.

Have your lenses checked regularly.

Regardless of whether you have hard or soft lenses, you should observe the following guidelines for your beauty-care program.

Don't use thin, runny day creams or night creams.

Don't apply cream too close to your eyes. Occasionally treat yourself to an eye mask when you don't have your lenses in.

Never apply eye cream all the way to the edge of the lid while wearing your lenses.

Don't use oily makeup.

Don't dust your face with loose powder while your lenses are in. It's too easy to get powder in your eyes. Use a compact and apply powder with a brush.

Always close your eyes while using hair spray or aerosol deodorants.

Use mascara and eye liner very carefully. They are major causes of eye irritation. Apply them after putting in your lenses. Don't use mascara applicators containing mink hair.

Don't apply eye liner to the top edge of your lower eyelid. Use liquid or cream eye shadow. Don't apply shadow too close to the lashes.

Take out your lenses before removing your makeup.

Insert contact lenses before applying makeup.

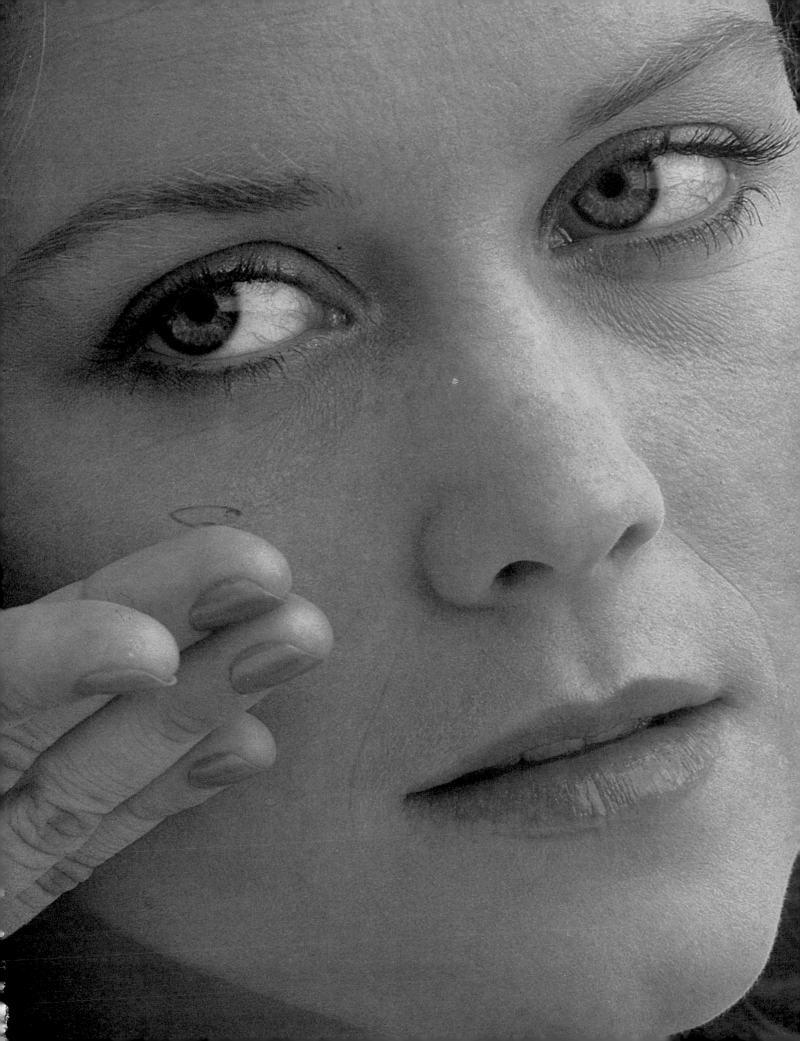

Makeup with Glasses

The right glasses should do more than improve your vision. They should complement your face. Their frames should enhance your facial structure. Their colors should match those of your eyes and hair.

Your eyebrows should be fully visible either over or under the top of the frames. Frames that cover part of your eyebrows look slightly out of proportion.

Don't choose a large frame if you have very thick lenses. Your glasses will be too heavy. They'll leave pressure marks on each side of your nose and will dig into the backs of your ears. They'll also tend to slide down.

If you're nearsighted, use eye makeup in dramatic colors.

Frames in natural colors, such as beige or eggshell white, are very flattering. Soft, translucent colors are also attractive.

Avoid black, dark-brown and tortoise-shell frames. They give your face a hard, old-fashioned look.

If you have pale skin, blemishes, or red, splotchy veins, avoid blue, purple, rust and green frames.

Glasses for everyday use are most flattering if they're inconspicuous. You should get them in neutral colors so they'll match all your clothing.

You should design your makeup with your glasses in mind. Wear dark, vibrant lipsticks. Apply blush more heavily than you would if you didn't have glasses.

Pay special attention to your eye makeup. If you're nearsighted, your glasses will make your eyes look smaller than they really are. Use light colors. Apply eye shadow more heavily at the outside corners of the eyes, and blend it up toward the brows.

Extend your eye liner slightly past the outside corners. Be sure to apply plenty of mascara—but do this carefully.

If you're farsighted, your glasses will make your eyes look larger. Avoid flashy colors and apply your makeup carefully. Dark eye shadow and highlighting cream and powder are not recommended. Use soft colors that match your skin tone. Eye liner should be applied only to the upper edge of the lower lid.

Glasses for farsighted people make their eyes look larger than they are. These glasses also magnify makeup mistakes.

Don't forget, groom your eyebrows very carefully. Untidy brows are much more noticeable behind glasses.

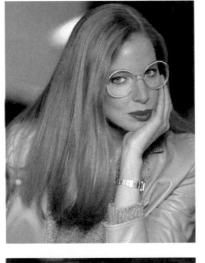

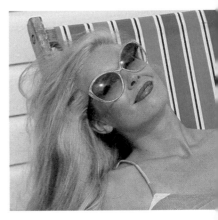

Good sunglasses involve more than beautiful frames. The lenses should be polarized to give you greatest protection from the sun.

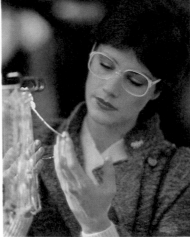

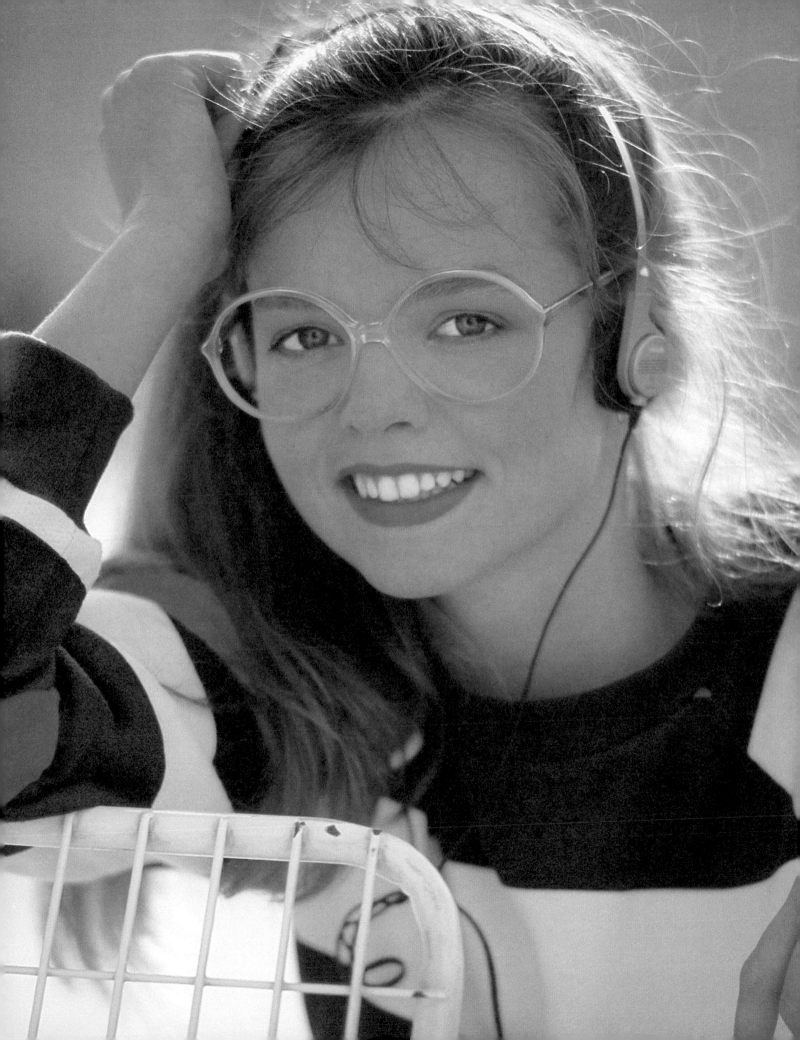

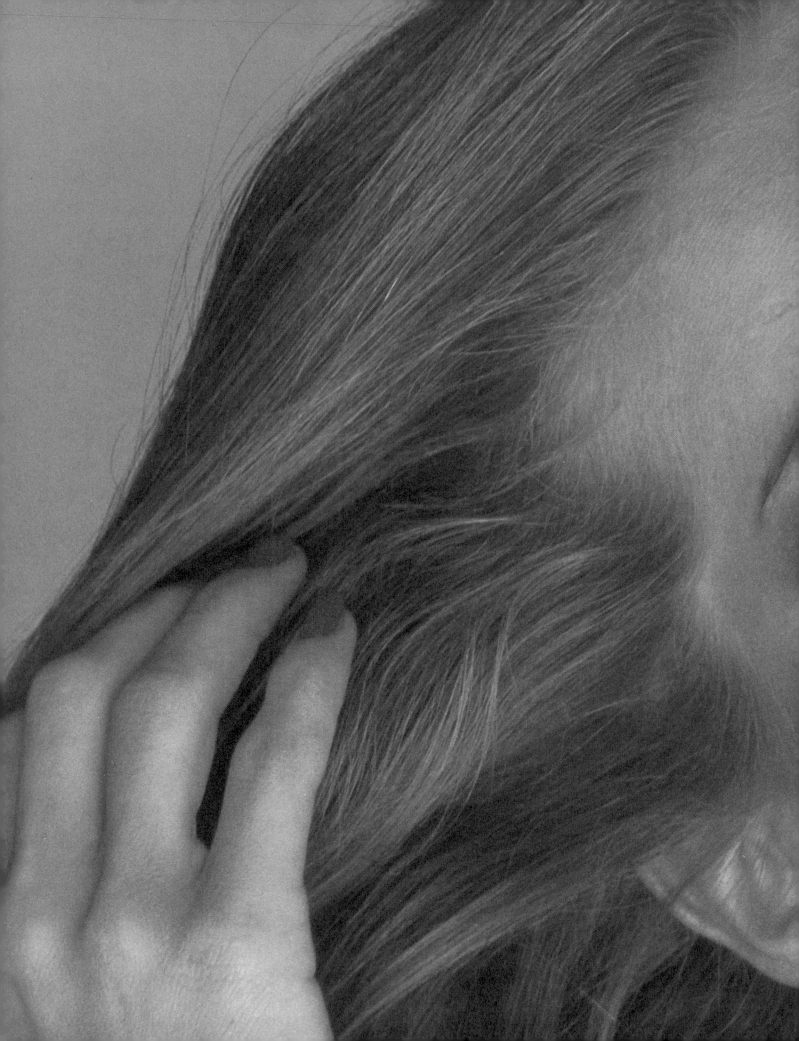

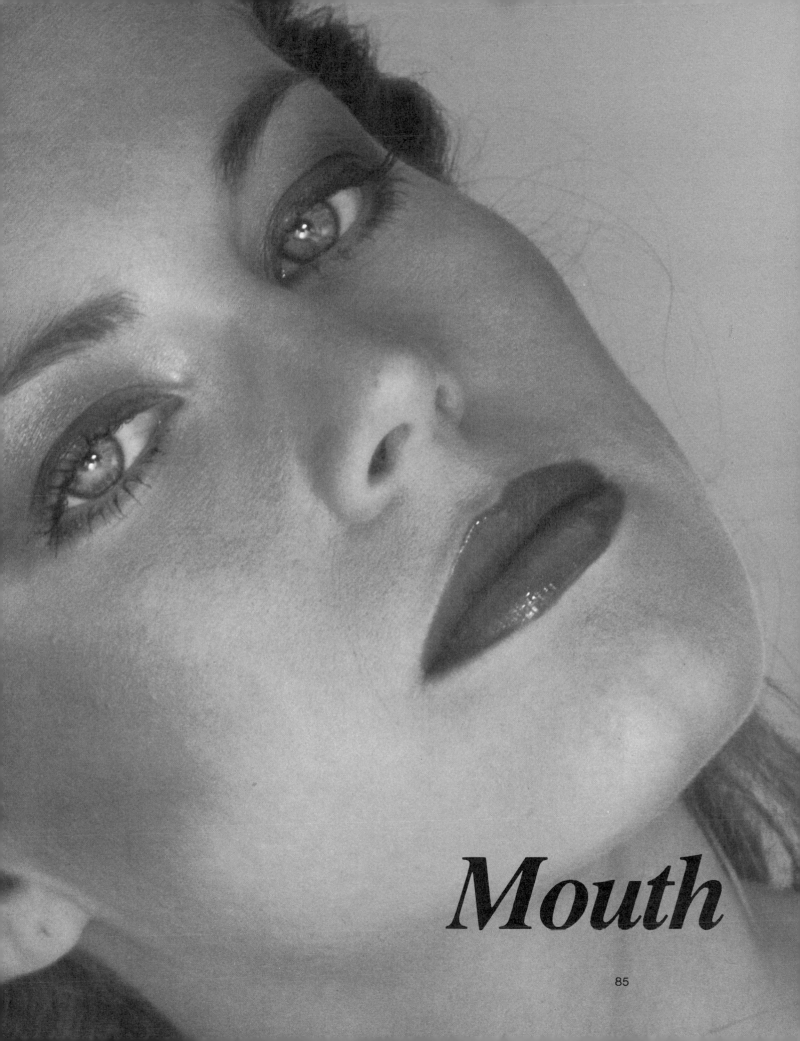

Mouth

Your mouth can be your most attractive facial feature. Use lipstick and gloss in appropriate colors to make it as beautiful as possible. You must also take care of your teeth, and that involves more than just brushing them. This chapter will show you the best techniques for putting the nicest possible smile on your face.

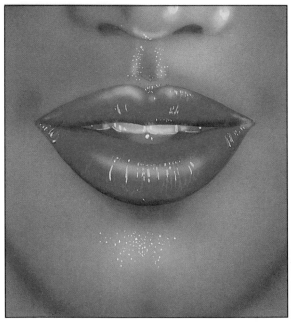

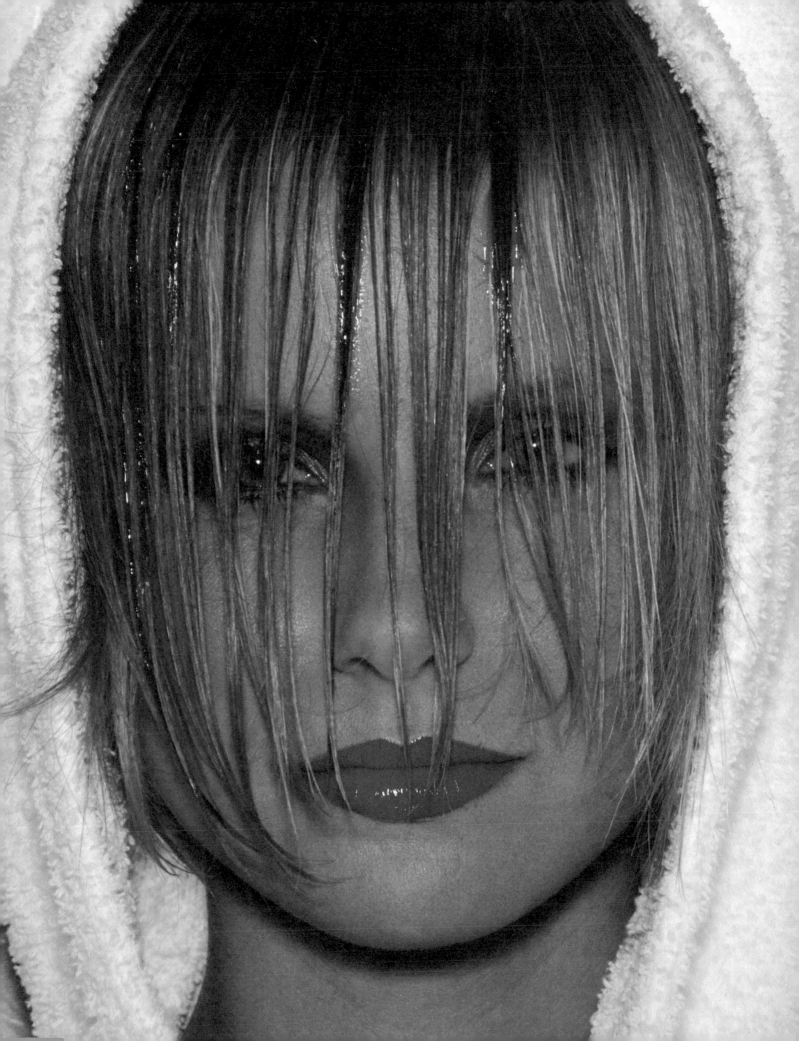

Makeup Techniques for Your Mouth

There are many ways to accentuate a pretty mouth or make a plain mouth more attractive. A perfectly made-up mouth catches the eye and diverts attention from other problems your face may have. It can make a large nose seem smaller, a pale complexion look livelier and blemishes appear less noticeable.

You'll get a good, sharp lip contour if you use a liner or pencil. These should be the same color as your lipstick or one shade darker. Don't use them to draw a straight line along your lip. Instead, dab them gently along the edge of your lip. Then blend the color in with the other end of the liner or pencil, or with your fingertip.

Don't use liner or pencil on the corners of your mouth. Your body heat will make the color you applied to the middle of your lips slightly moist, and it will flow gradually to the corners.

___

Buy lipsticks that are slightly sloped at the tip. You can apply them more precisely than lipsticks that are rounded.

___

If you use liner or pencil, apply lipstick with a brush. It will keep you from smudging the contours. Another advantage of a brush is that it enables you to use all the lipstick in your case. Usually a fifth of your lipstick lies below the rim of the case. You can't get it out without a brush.

___

Don't try to change the shape of your mouth too much with makeup. It will look unnatural.

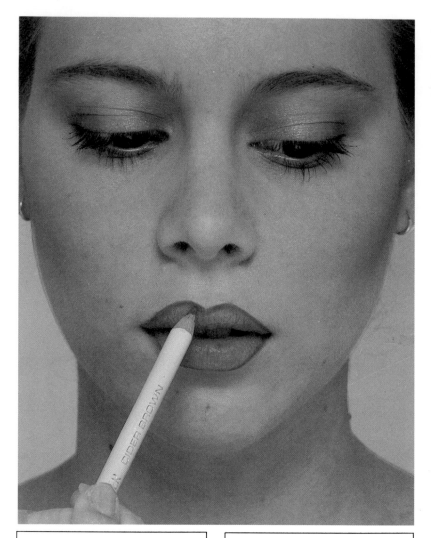

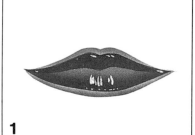 1

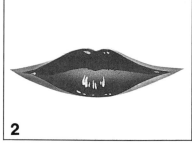 2

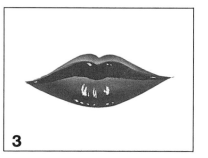 3

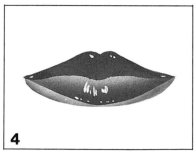 4

Your lip makeup will last longer if you blot your lipstick on a piece of tissue and then apply a second coat. Be sure not to use too much lipstick. It will rub off on your teeth and spoil your entire look.

The one thing you should never try with lip makeup is to alter the basic shape of your mouth. It looks ridiculous. If you want to make minor

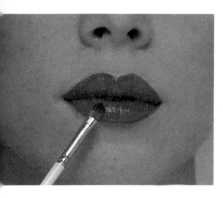

changes, apply foundation to your face and mouth first. This will make your lip color blend with your skin tone. It will also keep your lipstick from changing color. Apply your lipstick over your foundation.

The pictures on the facing page show you what to do.

Picture 1

If your lips are too small, apply liner or pencil to the outer edges. Don't go too far outside the natural lip line. Fill in your lips with a lipstick in a strong color. Put lip gloss on top of the lipstick. It makes your mouth look much fuller.

Picture 2

If your lips are too wide, use liner or pencil on the inner edges. Be sure not to extend the line to the corners of your mouth.

Picture 3

If your upper lip is too small, contour the inner edge of your lower lip.

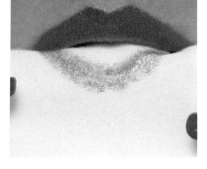

Picture 4

If your lower lip is too wide, contour only the upper lip. Don't use lipstick in bold colors and don't apply lip gloss.

The shape of your mouth isn't the only factor that determines which lipstick colors are best for you. Your hair color, complexion and clothes must also be considered.

If you have light hair and a light complexion, use soft colors. If your skin and hair are darker, use brighter, deeper colors.

If you don't want to change lipsticks with every fashion trend, choose a neutral color. Lipsticks with brown or pink tones work best.

Use very light lipstick only if your teeth are very white. Dark colors make teeth that are slightly gray or yellow appear lighter. Light colors make them appear darker.

After applying lipstick, press your lips on a tissue. Then apply another coat. This technique will make your mouth look prettier longer.

Makeup for Your Mouth

Cream lipsticks, translucent lipsticks, lip gloss, liquid lip makeup—the choice of lip products seems endless. Which ones will work best for you is not just a question of fashion. It also depends on the condition of your lips and the effect you want to create. Cream lipsticks are a good choice if you want a simple, straightforward look. They cover well because they have plenty of pigment.

Put honey on chapped lips. It provides immediate relief.

Translucent lipsticks look natural. They leave a translucent color film on your lips. They are also good for dry lips because they contain more oils. Translucent lipsticks do not look good with flashy makeup.

Lip gloss, which you can put on top of lipstick, gives your lips a very intense shine.

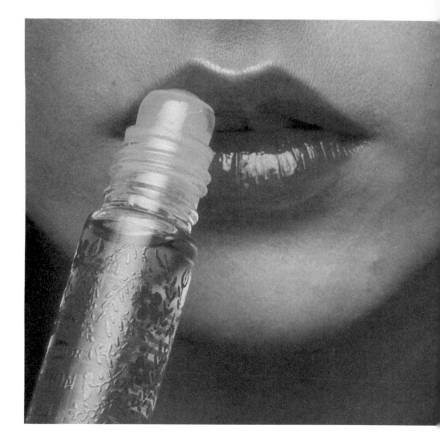

If you have chapped lips, use lip balm under your lipstick.

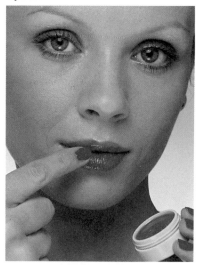

Most gloss is either colorless or slightly tinted. It is also beneficial for dry lips.

If you have very prominent lips, use gloss rather than lipstick. Try gloss containing mother-of-pearl.

If you use light gloss, dab it on with your fingertip. If you prefer dark-tinted gloss, apply it with a brush.

Liquid lip makeup, which comes in a container with a brush, covers very well. It is also handy because you can keep your fingers clean.

Crayons are a new cosmetic product that can be used in place of lip liner or lip pencil. They have the soft head of a lipstick, yet can be sharpened to a fine point.

Dark hair on your upper lip will kill the effect of the most beautiful mouth. You should bleach it or remove it with a depilatory cream or lotion.

If you decide to use

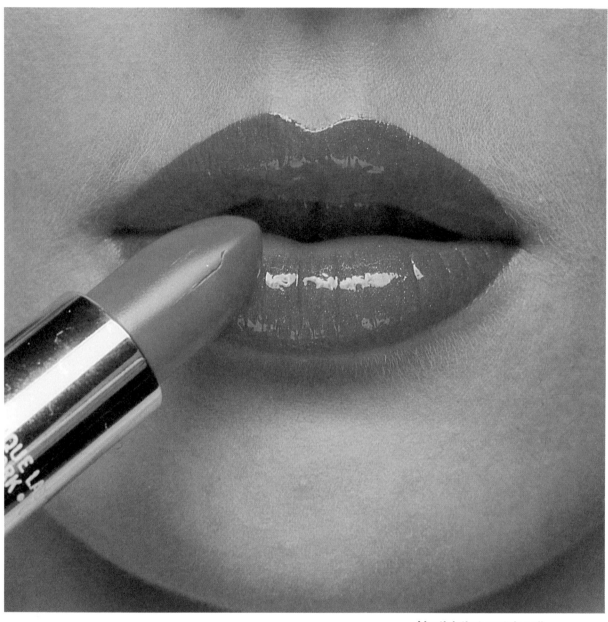

Lipstick that contains oil protects your lips from the elements.

bleaching cream, test your skin for allergic reaction first. Dab a little cream on the inside of your arm. Remove it after the recommended waiting time. If your skin doesn't become red or itchy within 30 minutes, you can use the cream on your face. Be sure to follow the directions on the package very carefully. The skin on your upper lip is very sensitive.

If you prefer using a depilatory, make the same test for allergic reaction beforehand. Put cream or lip balm on your lips before applying the depilatory to your face.

You'll have to use a bleaching cream or depilatory every 10 days to 2 weeks. You can only eliminate unwanted hair permanently through electrolysis. This procedure, which has to be done by an experienced professional, kills the hair follicles. It requires numerous sessions, and is expensive and somewhat painful.

Caring for Your Teeth

To have healthy teeth, you have to make sure they are always clean. Brush them after every meal if you can.

The proper brushing technique is important. Brush the front and back surfaces with downward strokes. Move from the gums all the way to the tips of your teeth.

Don't brush these surfaces of your teeth sideways. You won't remove plaque and will wedge food particles between your teeth. You can use sideways strokes only on the chewing surfaces.

Sugarless chewing gum helps keep breath fresh and won't promote tooth decay.

Your toothbrush should have short, rounded, artificial bristles. They are more hygienic than natural bristles. Be sure the bristles are soft. Hard bristles can damage gums. Replace your toothbrush every 2 to 3 months.

Electric toothbrushes move their bristles up and down automatically. Some of these brushes move with rough, rapid motions that can irritate your gums. Choose a brush that moves slowly and gently. This will set up a soft vibration that will massage your gums.

Be sure to use toothpaste with fluoride. This helps harden tooth enamel and prevent cavities.

Irrigating devices, which send streams of water between your teeth, can cleanse your mouth thoroughly and massage gums. However, some of these devices are too powerful. A forceful stream of water can break down gum tissue, which can lead to irritation and infection. It can also damage caps and bridges.

You should always carry dental floss and toothpicks in case you can't brush your teeth after meals. You should use floss at home at least once a day, even if you can't feel any food particles between your teeth. It cleans areas that your toothbrush can't reach.

Use toothpicks and floss carefully. They can irritate your gums.

It's very important to have regular dental checkups. Your teeth should be cleaned at least every 6 months to prevent plaque buildup and cavities.

Mouthwash cleanses and refreshes your mouth and throat.

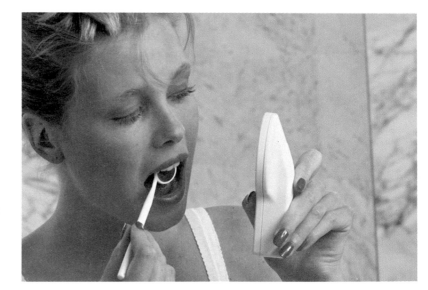

Many tools are available to help you take care of your teeth and gums. This small dental mirror is one of them.

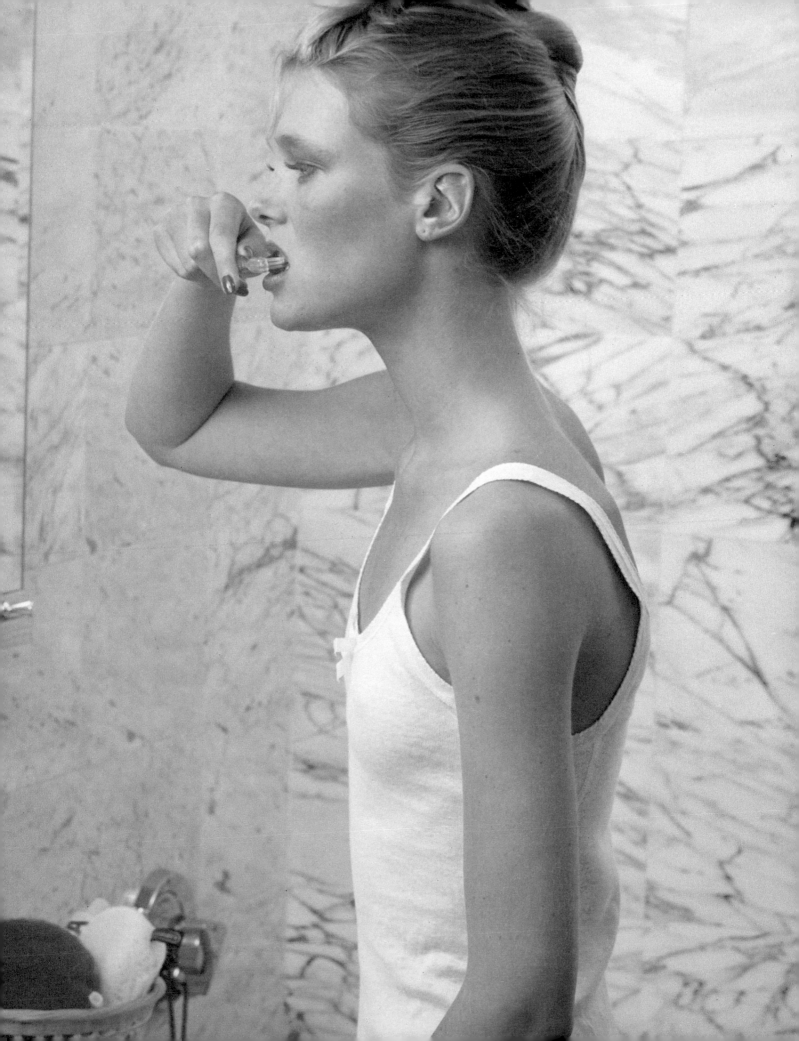

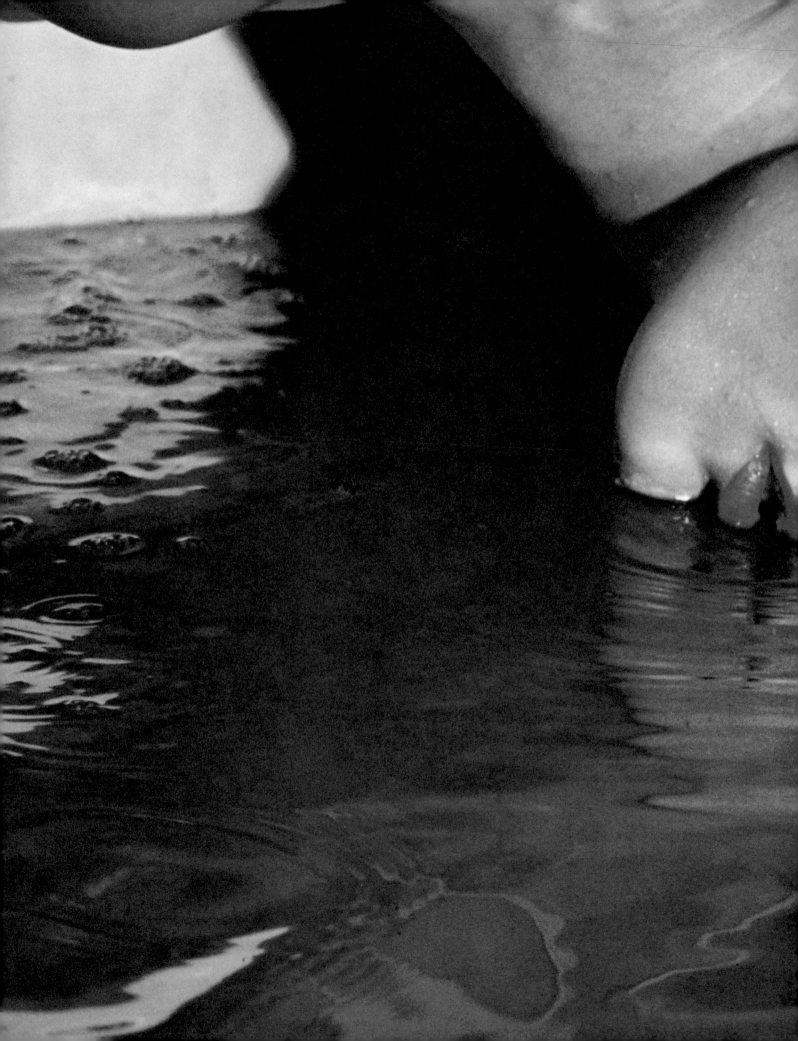

How to Apply Facial Makeup

Your complexion should appear fresh and rosy. The skin should have an even tone, and should be free of blemishes, irritation and pigment spots. Makeup can help your complexion look this way. Start by applying the right foundation for your skin type. Then put on powder to give your skin a soft, smooth look. Add blush. This cosmetic is like magic. It can make a square face appear rounder and can make a long face look shorter. Makeup can help 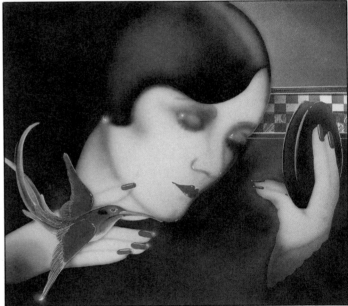 with other problems, too. Special products for troubled skin can help clear up blemishes and prevent pimples. Makeup for oily skin absorbs excess moisture. Cosmetics for dry skin are enriched with oil. Remember that applying makeup isn't an art. It's a series of easy-to-learn techniques.

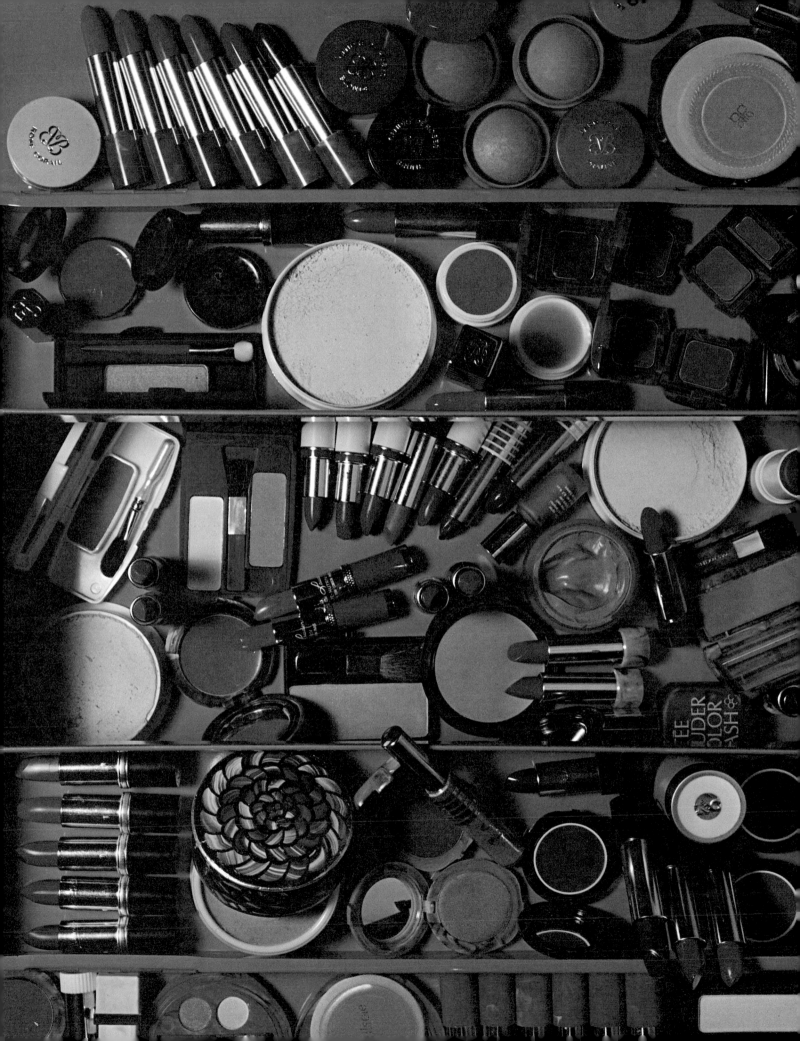

Foundation

Foundation makes your skin look even and supple. It covers blemishes and inflammation. Foundation also helps protect skin against the elements and pollution.

Your foundation should be about the same color as your complexion. If foundation is too dark, it makes you look older. It can also make your skin appear spotted.

Foundation that matches your skin is also easier to blend into your neck.

For dramatic effect, use makeup with glitter when you go out in the evening.

Before using foundation, you have to do several preliminary steps. First, cleanse your face and put on day cream or moisturizer. This gives your skin additional protection and helps you apply foundation smoothly and evenly.

Then cover dark circles under your eyes, pressure marks from glasses and tiny red veins with concealer. Cover blemishes with an antiseptic cream or lotion. These products should be slightly lighter than the foundation.

You can cover dark circles under your eyes with concealer. Use it before applying foundation. If you have blemishes, cover them with antiseptic cream or lotion.

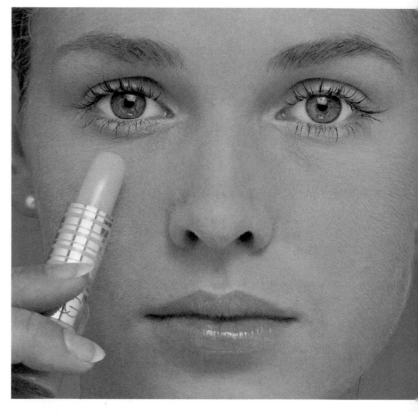

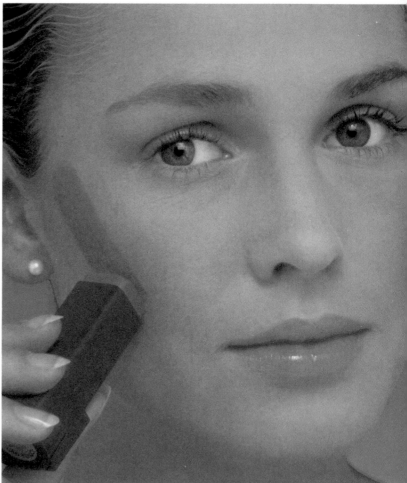

If you use a thick, creamy foundation, it will look more natural if you apply it with a little sponge. Moisten the sponge with water, then wring it out well. Spread a little foundation on the sponge, then squeeze it. Gently rub it on your face with small, circular motions.

If you use a thin, translucent foundation, apply it with your fingertips. Remember that this type of foundation will not conceal blemishes or pigment spots.

After several hours, perspiration and skin oil will make your foundation slightly streaked or spotty. Press tissues gently against your face to absorb the excess moisture.

Don't forget to blend the edges of your makeup into your neck.

Then lightly dust your face with powder from your compact. Don't apply more foundation. It will give your face a masklike effect.

If you don't like to wear makeup during your leisure time or if you have flawless skin, you can use a tinted cream instead of foundation. Tinted day creams enhance the natural color of your skin and make it appear fresh and moist. Tinted creams contain almost no pigment, so they don't conceal facial flaws.

If you're going to participate in water sports, use waterproof gel instead of foundation. Put a little on a cotton ball and smooth it over your skin with swift, circular motions. These gels tend to get spotty if they aren't applied quickly.

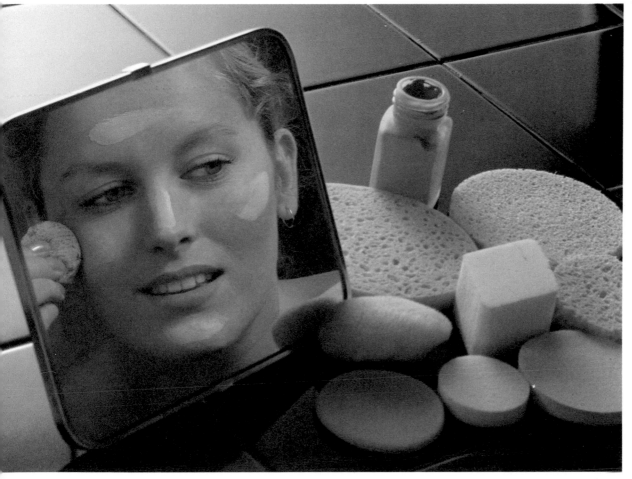

Your foundation will look more even and natural if you apply it with a sponge. The one exception is translucent foundation. You should apply this with your fingertips.

Powder

Powder gives your makeup a finished look. It makes skin look soft. You can buy loose powder or pressed compact powder. You should carry compact powder in your purse. It's very practical for touch-ups. But this type of powder contains very few moisturizers, so skin tends to get oily.

Loose powder looks prettier longer. It is very translucent and lies on your skin like a fine veil if applied properly. Dip your brush or puff lightly into the powder. Dab the brush or puff several times on the palm of your hand to get rid of the excess. Pat it over your skin with quick, delicate movements. Remove excess powder from your face with a powder brush. Use downward strokes so your facial hair will continue to lie flat.

If you have a good, even complexion and want a natural look, apply powder over your day cream. Tissue off excess day cream before using the powder. Don't use foundation at all.

Some dermatologists also recommend this technique if you have oily skin.

If you start to perspire on your forehead or upper lip, don't wipe off perspiration with your powder puff. This is not good for your skin and makes your complexion look spotty. Use tissue to remove the perspiration, then carefully reapply powder.

Brushes and puffs should always be clean. You don't have to buy new ones when they begin to get oily. Just wash them with a mild detergent.

Powder puff or brush? You can use either with loose powder. If you would rather use the puff, remove excess powder from your face by brushing with downward strokes.

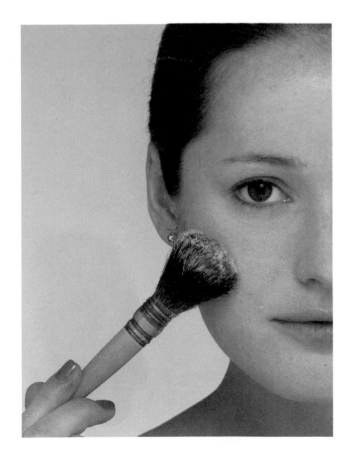

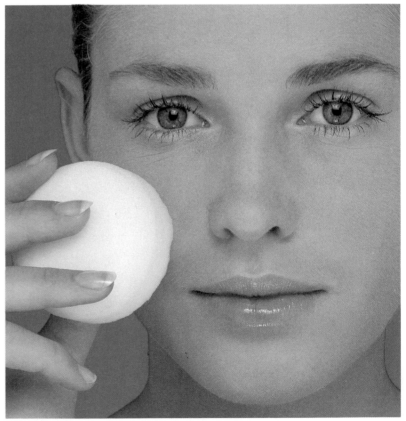

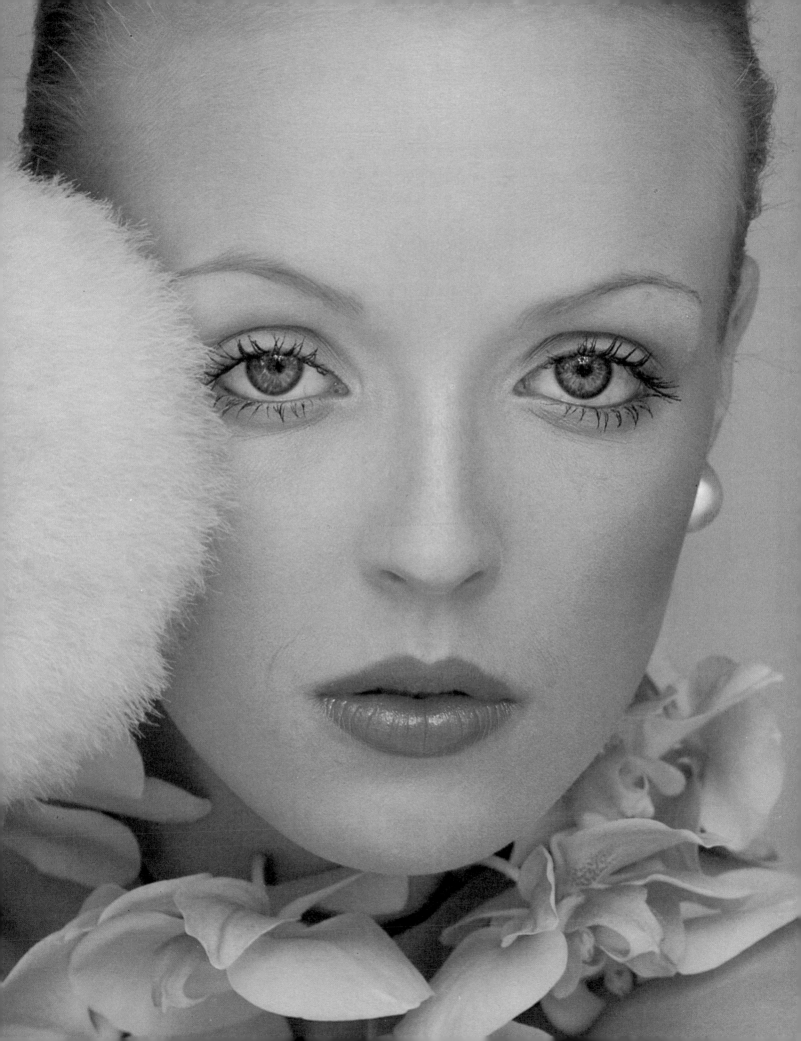

Blush

You should not use cream or liquid blush if you have fine hair on your forehead and cheeks. These products make facial hair much more noticeable. Blush sticks and powder are effective for everyone. These products are also easy to carry in your purse.

To use blush, put a small streak of color on each cheekbone. Then blend it in well. Use a sponge with cream or liquid blushes, and a brush with powder. Your fingertips work best with blush sticks.

Blush should look understated and natural. If you use too much, it will look as if you've painted red spots on your face.

Blush can make your face look longer or rounder, depending on how you apply it.

If you have a round face, put blush in the middle of your cheekbone. Blend it back toward the hairline in a triangle. The base of the triangle should extend from the cheekbone to the middle of your earlobe.

With a square face, apply blush in the middle of your cheekbone and blend it in a straight line along the bone.

If you have a triangular face, put blush high on your cheekbone and blend it back toward your hairline in a small triangle.

To shorten a long face, put blush on the outside of your cheeks, toward the base of your cheekbone. Blend it back, following the curve of the cheekbone.

Gold powder on your cheeks looks especially attractive in the evening. You can apply it instead of blush or on top of blush.

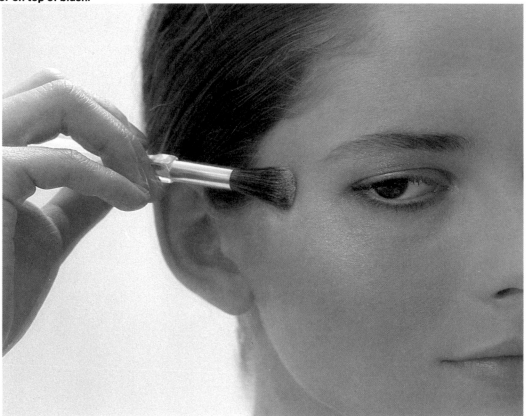

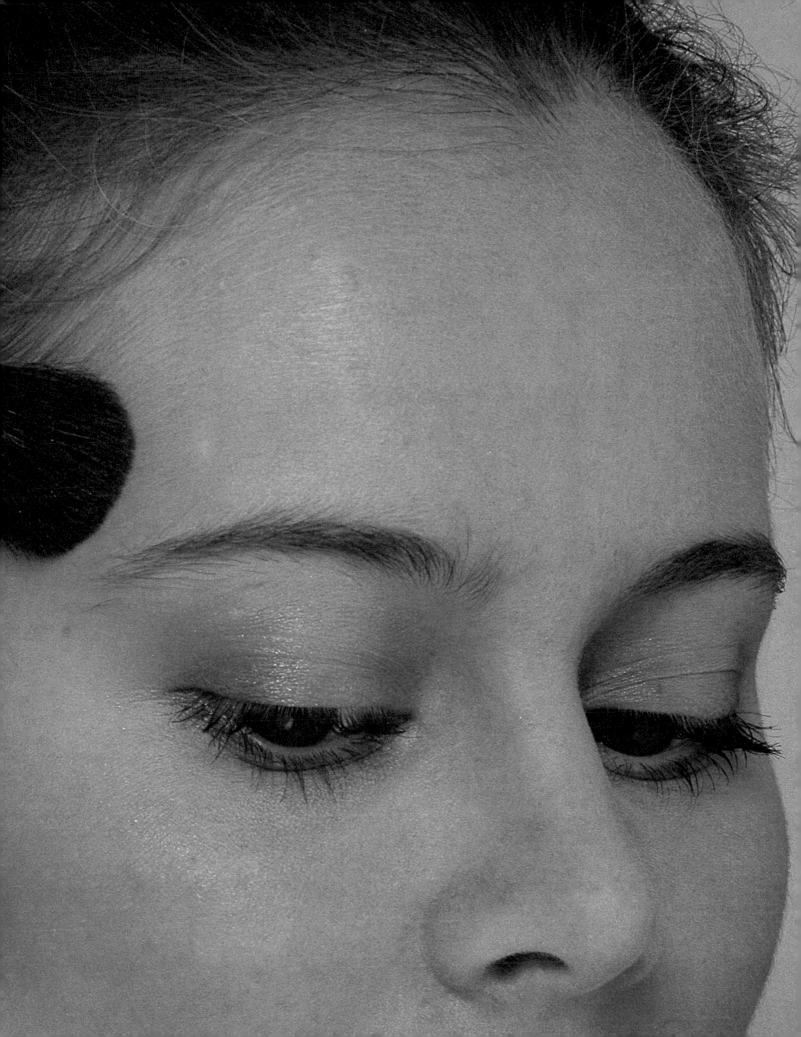

Choosing the Right Colors

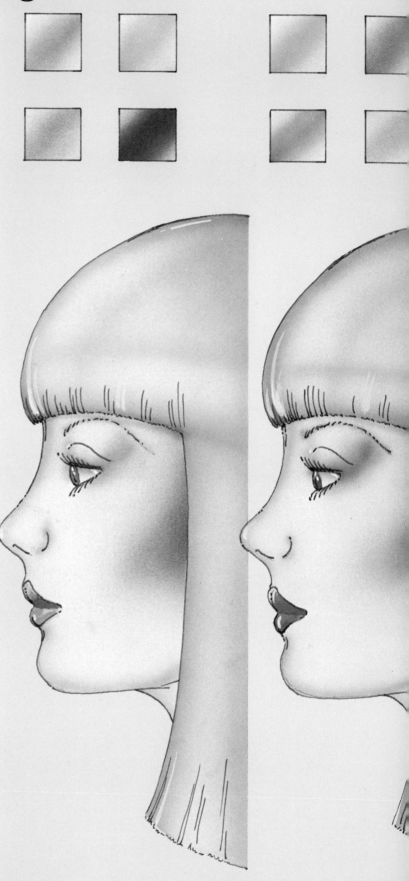

Your makeup colors will depend principally on your hair and eye colors. Fashion trends and clothes should also play a minor part in your deliberations.

Light blondes should use only very light colors. Eyebrows should be light brown or gold. Medium blondes should use colors that are a shade darker. Blondes can use even darker colors if they have a tan.

Women with light brown hair usually have very pale skin. They need plenty of blush.

If you're pale, don't try to compensate with dark foundation. Use blush instead.

Redheads look most attractive in shades ranging from orange to rust. Soft blues and greens are also attractive.

Brunettes get best results with sand-colored foundation. Colors for eyes, lips and blush can be stronger.

Women with black hair should use soft, light colors.

If you're unsure about which colors look best on you, use eye shadow, blush and lipstick that are a shade lighter than you think they should be. It's always better to have colors that are a little too light rather than a little too dark.

The small colored squares show you which lipstick, blush and eye shadow colors match your hair color.

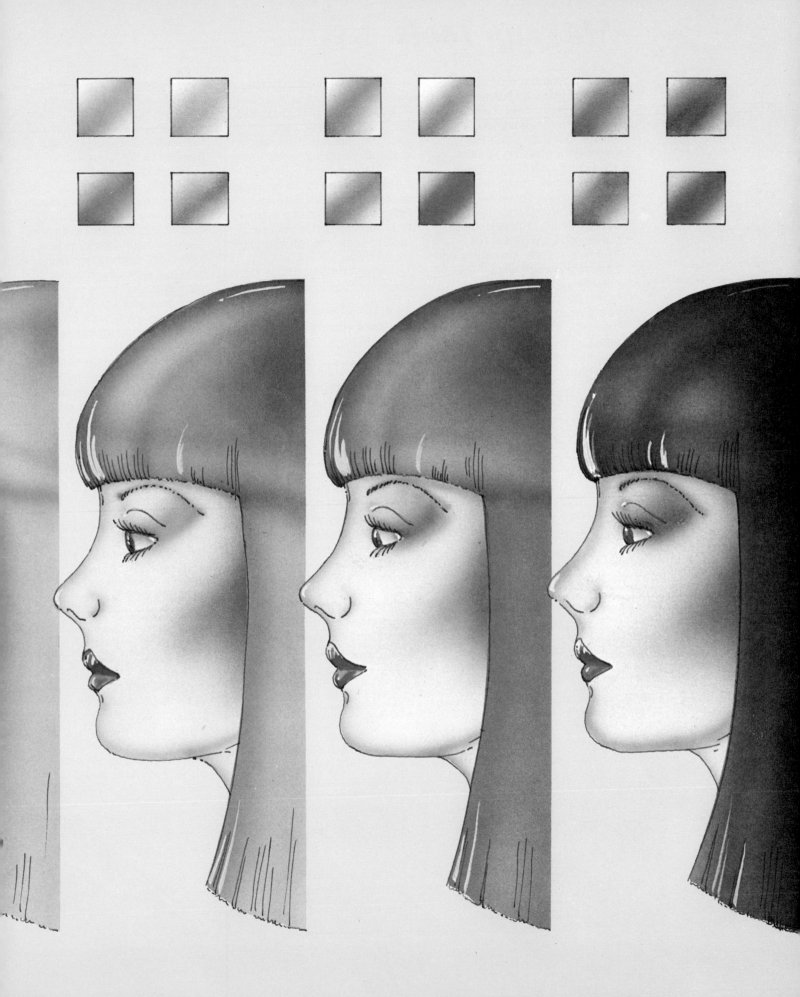

Makeup Tools

If you're going to apply makeup properly, you must have the right tools. The most important item is a good mirror. One side should have magnifying glass, so you can get a close look as you apply your eye liner and lip liner.

For eye care you'll need tweezers, an eyebrow brush, an eyelash brush, an eyelash curler and a sharpener for eyebrow pencils. You may also have to buy applicators for eye shadow and liquid eye liner.

For the rest of your face, you'll need sponges for foundation, a powder puff, a powder brush and a compact. Brushes are usually included with blush.

Always have cotton swabs and tissues on hand.

Having the right light is also important when you are applying makeup. If you put makeup on during the day, you should use natural light. You might apply too much makeup otherwise, because artificial light has a reddish or greenish tint. Makeup that looks fine indoors looks orange when you step outside.

To apply makeup properly, you need the right tools and the right lighting.

Another problem is that lights above or on the sides of mirrors tend to cast shadows. Makeup that looks fine in this light looks harsh and unnatural outdoors.

For best results, apply your makeup while sitting by a window, facing the light.

If you can't do this, be sure to check your makeup once you leave the house to be sure it doesn't look too bright or garish.

If you're going out in the evening, you'll have to apply makeup under artificial light. If you're going to a place with neon light, use very soft colors.

Bright makeup can easily make you look old and hard under this type of light. You'll get a good idea of how your makeup will look if you apply it under fluorescent light.

Wherever you put on your makeup, remember to have light shining in the mirror from behind you. Light from the side accentuates wrinkles and pores. Light from above makes you look older. It brings out the bags and dark circles under your eyes and the lines around your nose and mouth. Even light from the front is better to use than light from the side or from above.

Several techniques will make you look lovelier in evening light. Try putting on powder, blush or eye shadow with glitter. If you're going to use these cosmetics, be sure to wear good foundation. When you apply these products, do so sparingly. A little glitter looks glamorous. Too much looks ludicrous.

You can also use highlighting cream or powder in silver, silver-rose or gold. Apply it very lightly with a brush, then remove the excess with a clean powder brush. A little liquid glitter cream can be very dramatic. You can easily apply it with your fingertips.

Lipstick with glitter can be a nice touch, but it looks best in very low light.

Be especially careful with these cosmetics if you have oily skin. They may simply make your face look oilier. Use glitter only on your lips, eyes and the outside of your cheeks.

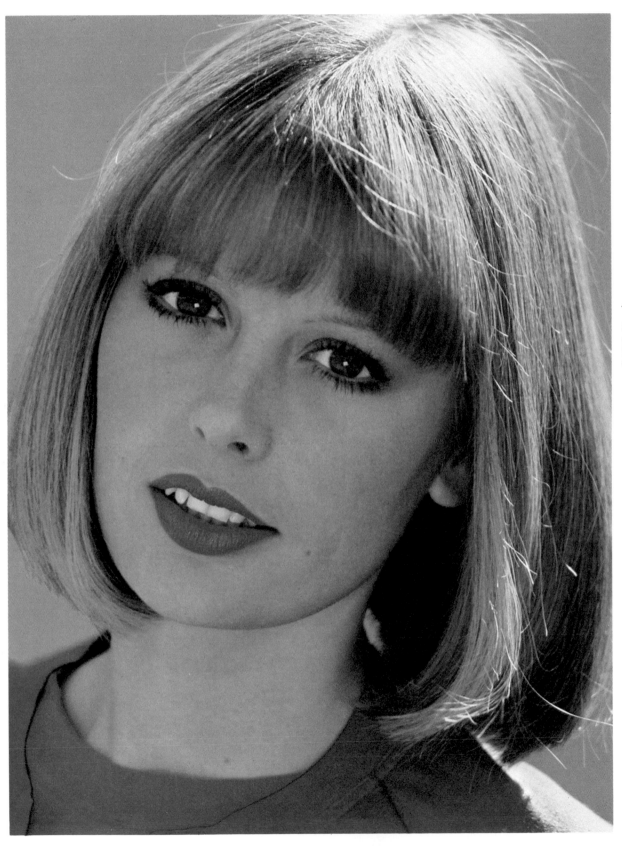

Sporty: A fresh look for every day. The bright lipstick is the most eye-catching feature.

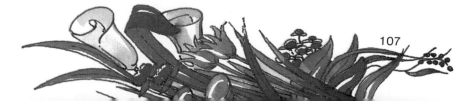

107

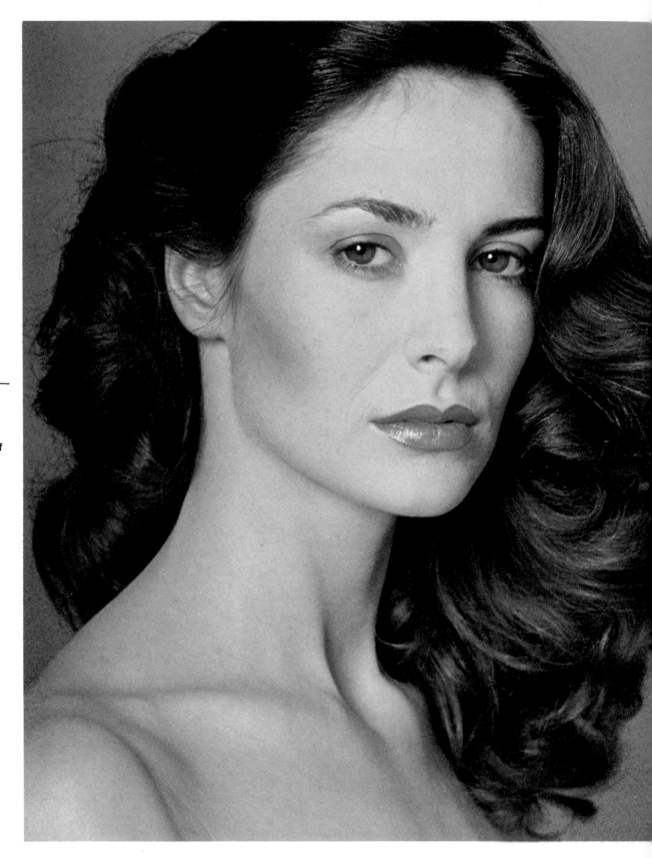

Classic: A timeless
look that brings out
the beautiful facial
features. The fine
translucent colors of
the lips and eyes
match the light
complexion.

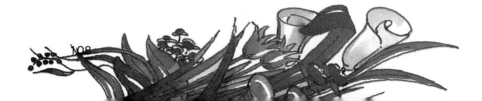

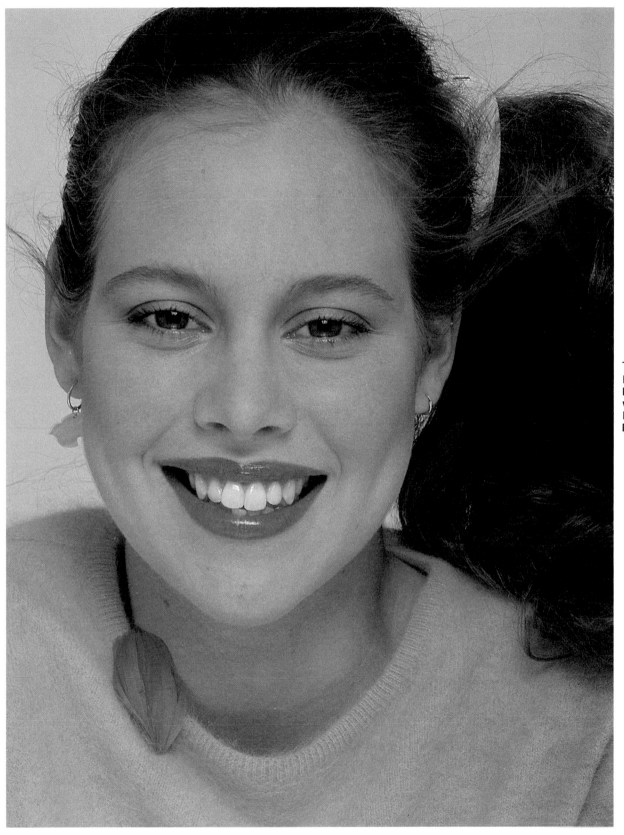

Natural: An understated look for those who don't want to appear made up. Blush and eye shadow have light brown tints.

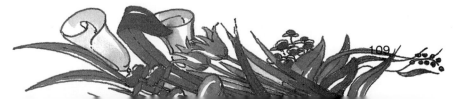

Elegant: An extravagant
look for special occasions.
Lips, cheeks and eyes are
pink and mauve,
complemented with gloss.

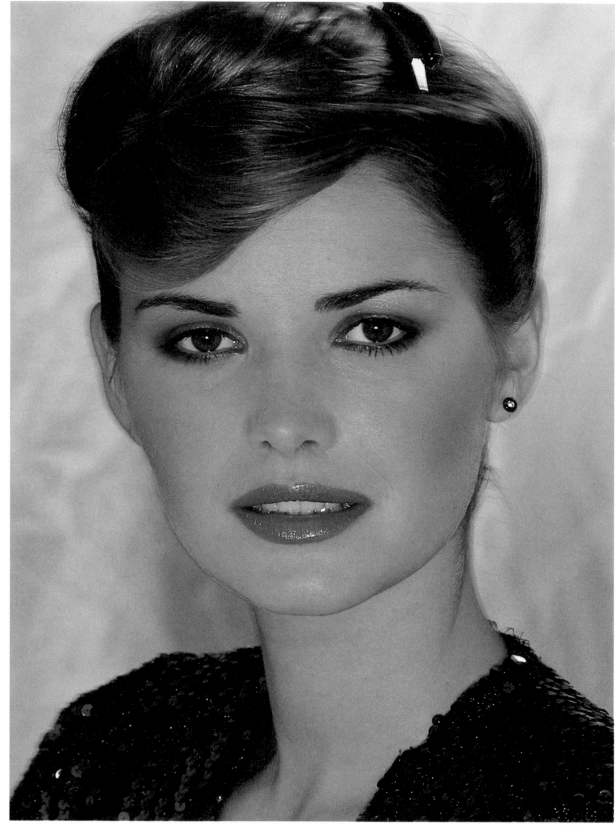

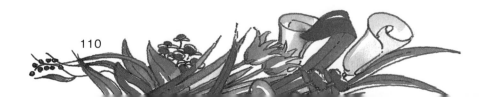

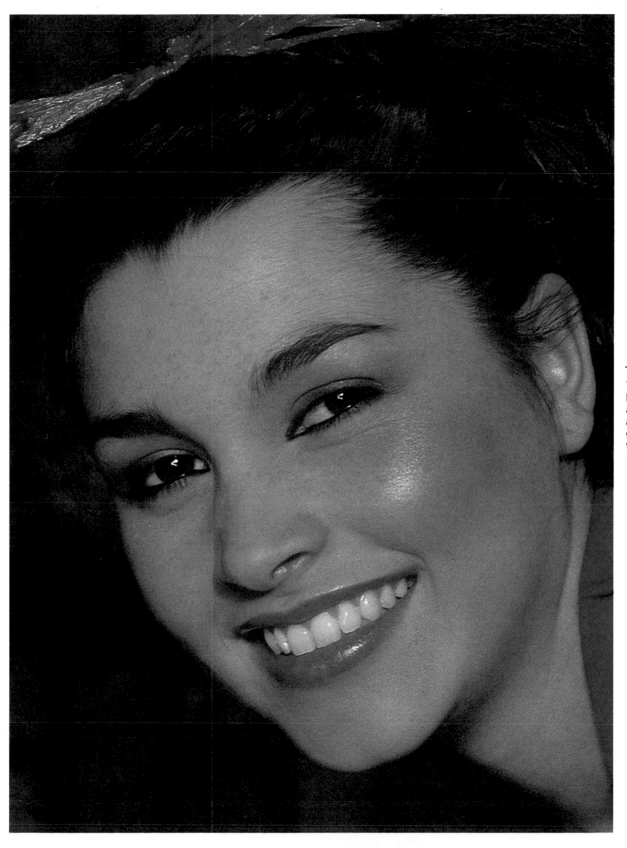

Youthful: A subtle look that is very alluring. Gold blush and rust-colored lip gloss go very well with the black eye liner.

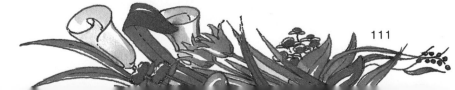

111

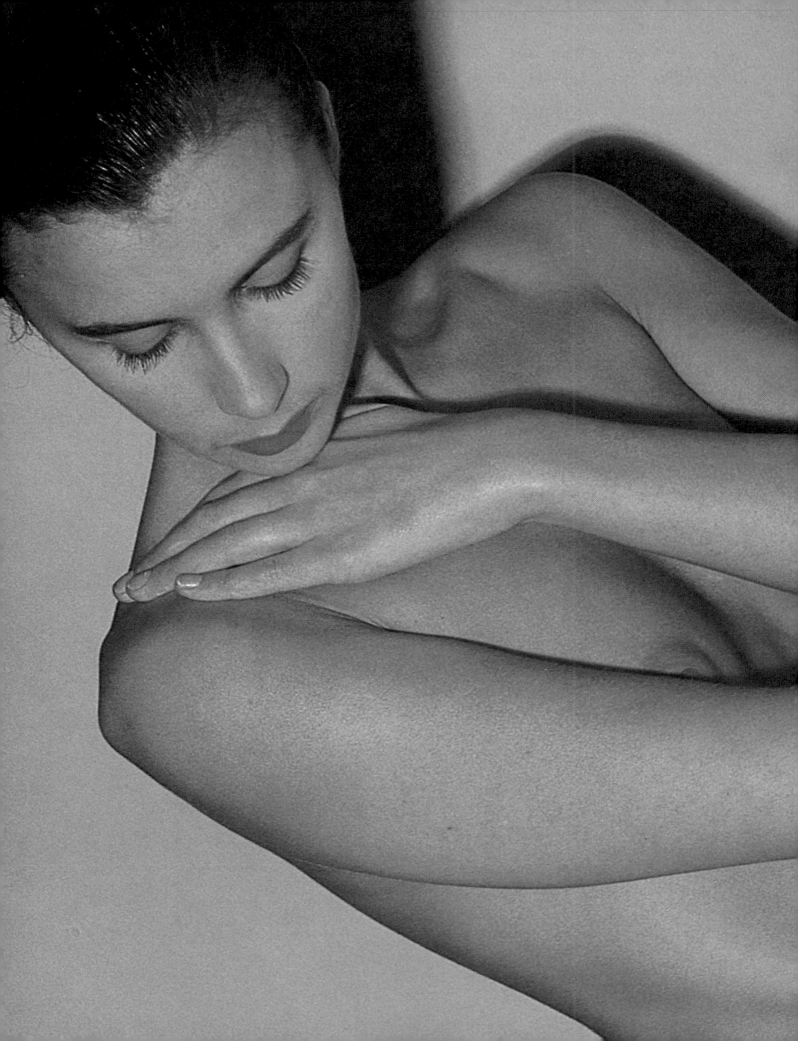

Shoulders, Arms, Breasts and Abdomen

Without a doubt you can hide your shoulders, arms, breasts and abdomen. But what if you occasionally want to wear a sleeveless blouse, a dress with a plunging neckline or a bikini? A more beautiful idea is to spend time taking care of these parts of your body. Exercise and massage them so skin and muscles don't lose elasticity. You must exercise regularly, preferably a few minutes each day. Watch your posture. Remember, chest out, stomach in, shoulders back. This is the best and least expensive beauty treatment. After bathing, be sure to apply body lotion or moisturizing cream. It will keep these areas smooth and soft. Then use dusting powder and light perfume.

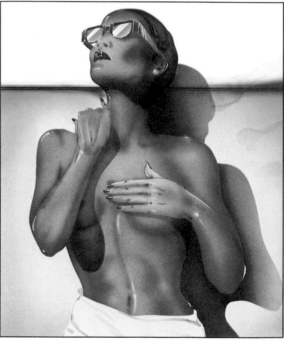

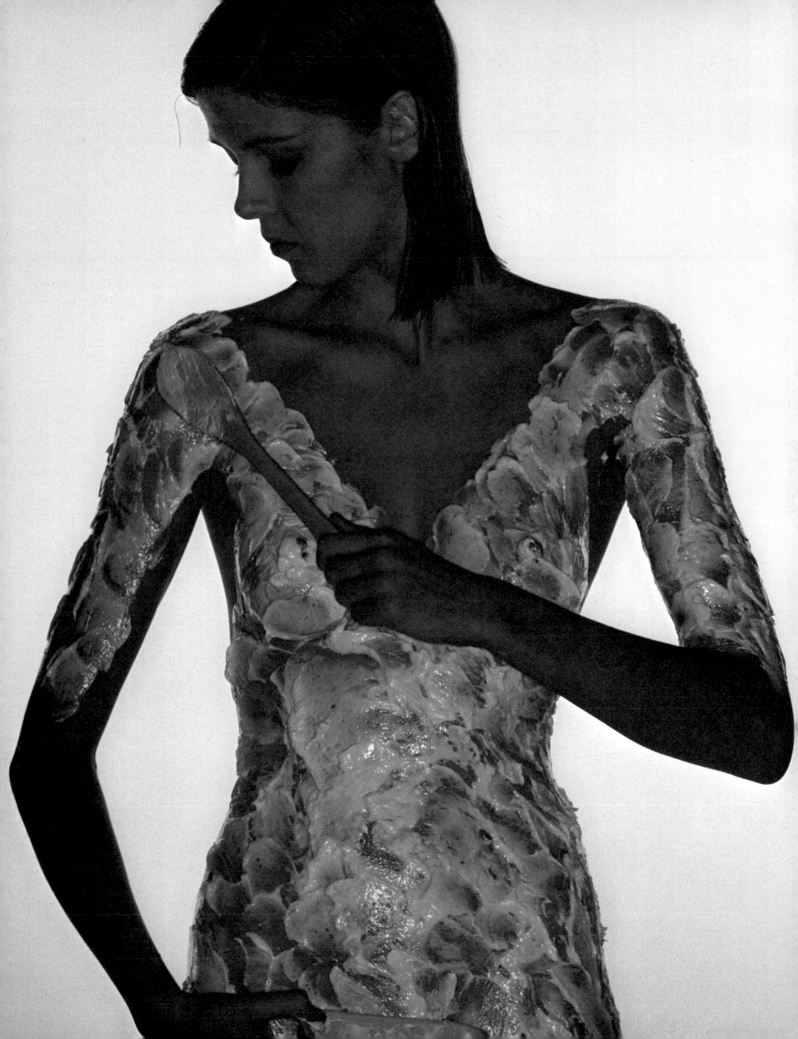

Shoulders and Arms

These areas can't be neglected if you want a well-groomed appearance. The first step is removing underarm hair. Hair-removing creams work best. You can also use wax, but it is somewhat painful and can burn you severely if not used properly. Shaving is not as effective, because armpits do not have an even surface. Stubble always remains and skin is easily cut or irritated. An electric shaver gives better results than a razor.

After removing hair, lightly powder your underarms. This minimizes irritation. Never use deodorants immediately afterward. Many contain alcohol and will irritate skin. The best time to remove hair is just before going to bed. Skin will be fine by morning.

You should massage your shoulders and arms every day with a body brush. Shower afterward to remove dead skin cells. Then use plenty of moisturizing cream. Shoulders look even more attractive with a touch of powder.

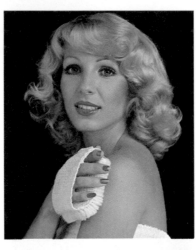

When you give your arms a beauty treatment, pay special attention to your elbows. No other part of your body is treated as roughly. Skin is often rough, cracked, even calloused. Massage your elbows after your daily shower or bath with a *loofah glove.* Then apply a body lotion with a high fat content.

If your elbows are very dry and calloused, soaking in a tub will help. Put warm body oil in two small bowls and soak your elbows for five minutes. Then rub them thoroughly with a pumice stone.

By the way, the beauty treatment you give your face will work very well on your elbows!

Shoulders and arms are often neglected because they are not typical female problem areas. You should massage these areas to ensure good circulation. You should also powder your shoulders and put moisturizing cream on your arms and elbows.

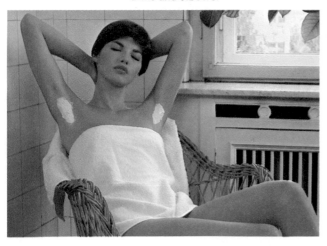

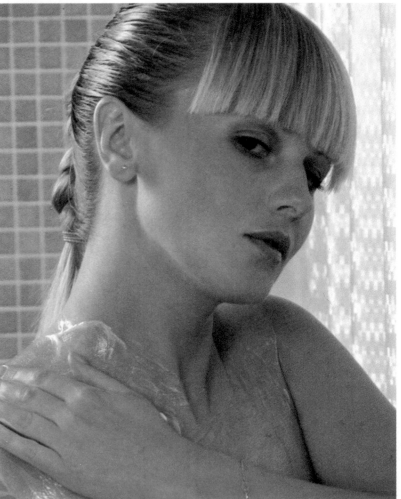

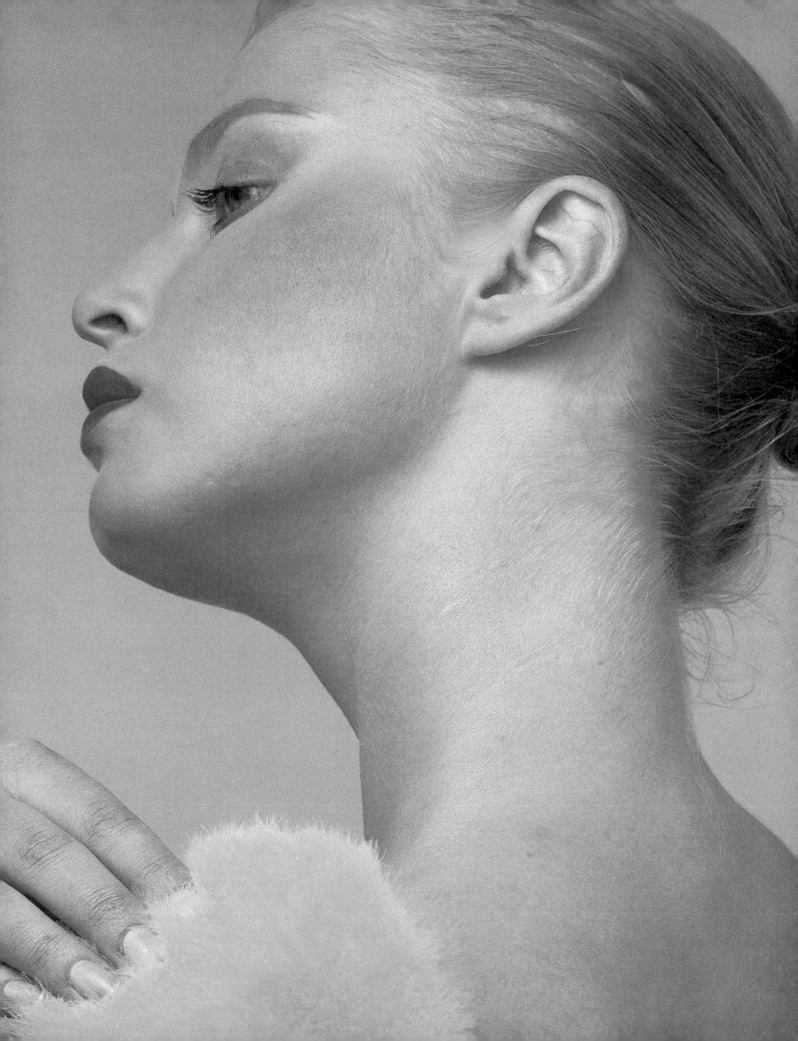

Upper Chest and Bosom

A pretty bust and upper chest are important, especially in summer, when you wear thin blouses and bathing suits. This part of your body has very sensitive skin and tissue. Daily care will keep it free of small blemishes.

Good circulation is essential. You can improve circulation by alternating hot and cold water in your shower. Be sure the water is not turned on full force. This can damage small veins.

If your bra is too tight, it will squeeze the skin between the breasts, making the skin look wrinkled.

Massage your upper chest each day with a loofah glove or body brush with fairly stiff bristles. Rub with a light, circular motion.

If your skin is too sensitive for this type of massage, apply a commercial facial scrub. It will help clear up blemishes and smooth rough spots.

You can keep the area around the collarbone pretty by massaging it with a brush and rinsing in cold water at the end of each shower.

After bathing and massaging, always cover the breasts and upper chest with a body lotion or moisturizer.

Daily exercise is a good way to improve breast tone. It strengthens the tissue and muscles underlying your breasts.

When you wear a low-cut dress or blouse, cover small blemishes with a concealing cream. Blend the edges. Don't use foundation. It will stick to your clothing.

Complete your beauty regimen by applying transparent powder from neck to breast. If you're going to a party or formal affair, put a touch of gold powder on the collarbone and upper chest.

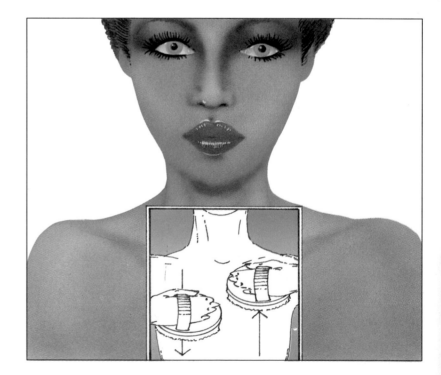

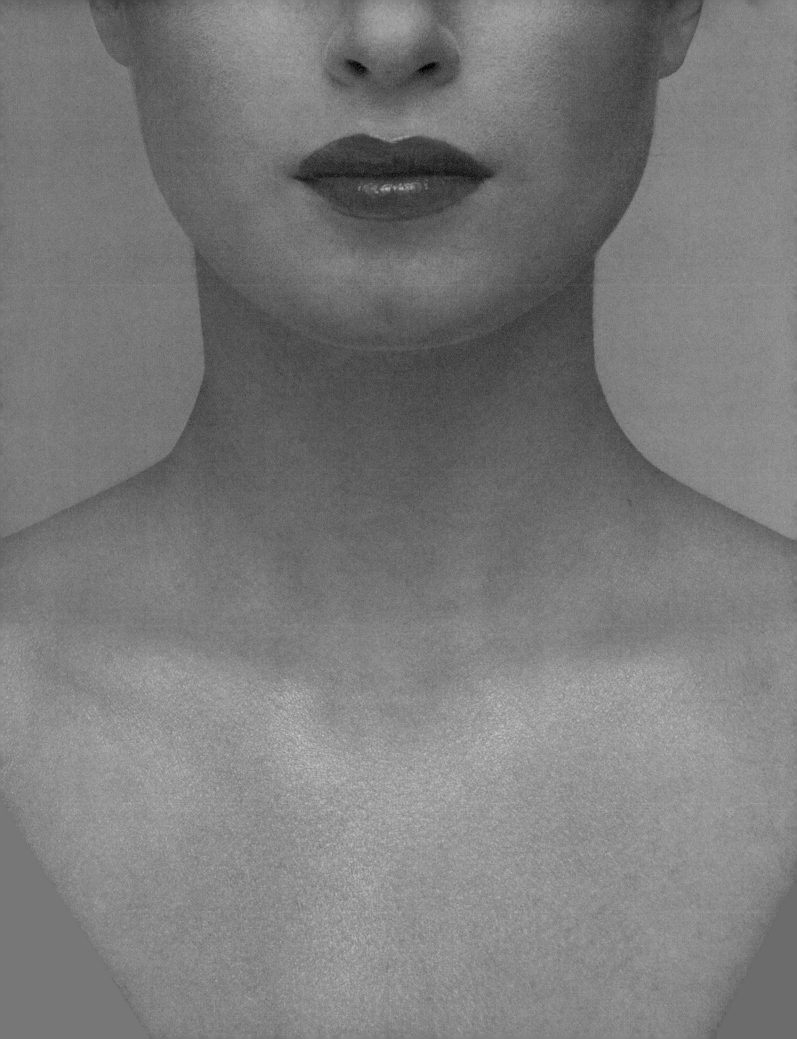

Breast Exercises

Remember that the size and shape of breasts are inherited. The best thing to do is accept this and learn to like the way you are. The only way to significantly change your breasts is through surgery. Even if you are willing to have an operation, think it over carefully first. Surgery is very expensive and results in permanent scars. Some women's breasts also lose sensitivity afterward.

You can strengthen the muscles underlying your breasts with exercises shown on these facing pages. You can significantly supplement these exercises by swimming, rowing, playing ball and lifting weights.

When you do any sustained exercise, be sure to warm up

Daily exercise and good posture help keep your breasts looking beautiful.

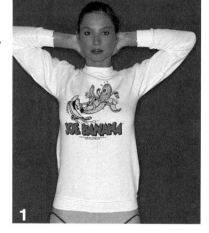

first. Spend at least 5 minutes doing stretches and slow, easy exercises. Warming up is crucial if you are going to do any exercise that will significantly increase your heart rate.

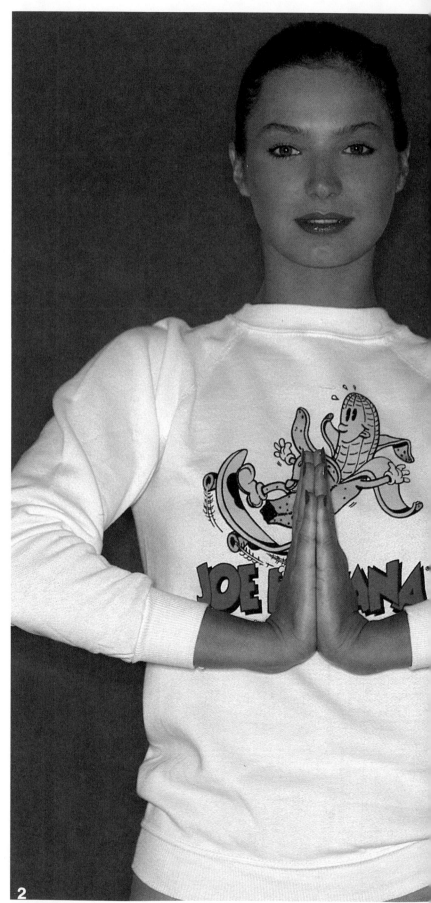

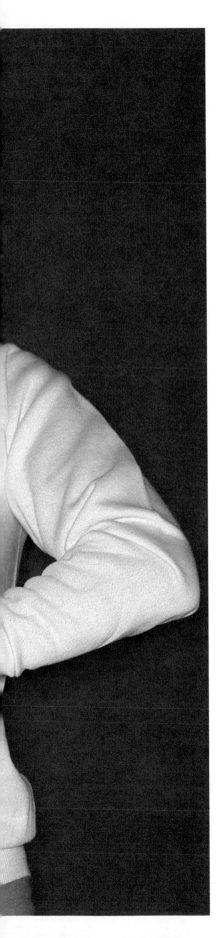

It is also important to cool down after exercising. Spend at least 5 minutes gradually reducing the intensity of your exercise to give your muscles an opportunity to relax. Stretching after strenuous exercise is also helpful.

You should exercise regularly at the same time of day. Don't look for excuses not to exercise. They are too easy to find.

This book will tell you how to have beautiful breasts without surgery. No matter what type of breasts you have—small, large, rounded, pointed—you can make them lovelier through exercise and proper skin care.

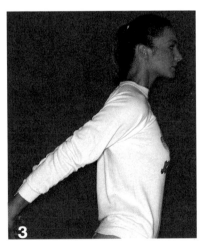

Persistence and patience are the keys. Only a daily, long-term program leads to lasting success. Doing something every 2 or 3 months accomplishes nothing.

Your beauty program must be designed to keep your skin tight and supple and to encourage muscle tone in the chest.

Picture 1

Stand straight. Clasp your hands behind your head. Pretend you are facing a stone wall and press your elbows forward, into the "wall," as hard as you can. This is an isometric exercise, so your arms and elbows should not actually move. Keep pressing elbows forward for 5 seconds. Relax. Repeat 15 times, working up to 30.

Picture 2

Place palms together in front of your chest. With elbows high, press palms firmly together. Hold 5 seconds, then relax. Repeat 10 times, working up to 30.

Picture 3

Stand relaxed, feet shoulder-width apart. Clasp your hands behind your back

You should do bust exercises every day.

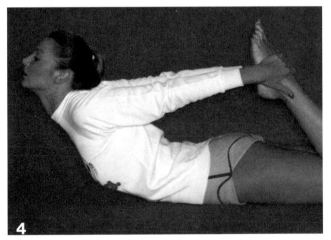

and straighten your arms. Your palms should be open and facing upward. Pull your arms quickly upward, as high as you comfortably can. Repeat 15 times, working up to 30.

Picture 4

Lie face down on the floor. Spread your legs slightly, bend your knees and grab your ankles. Lift your head, chest and thighs as high as you can. Hold 3 seconds, then relax. Repeat 5 times, working up to 15.

Stomach and Waist Exercises

Are you not really heavy, just out of shape? Do you have difficulty stopping yourself when you start overeating? Do you have unattractive fat rolls instead of elegant curves? Then do something about it, starting now!

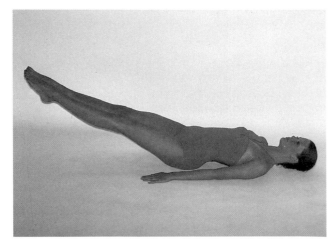

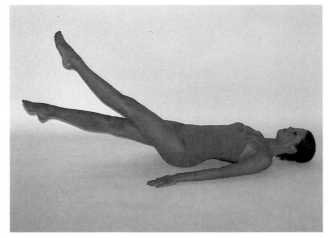

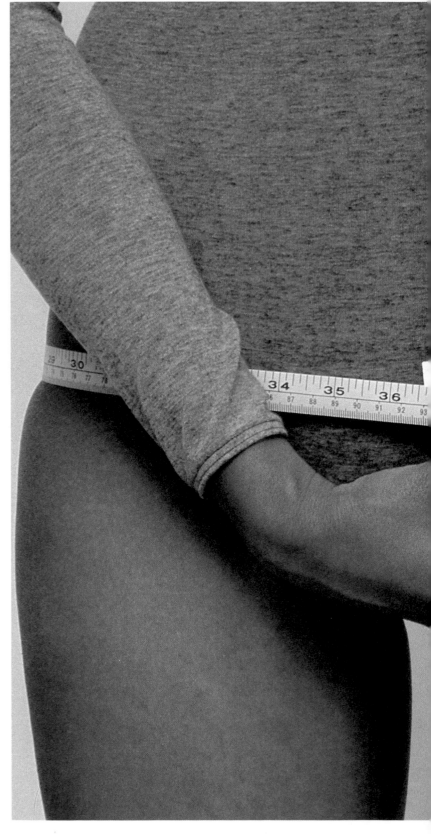

Here is a special exercise to flatten and firm your stomach. Lie on the floor. Straighten and lift your legs about 18 inches off the floor. Lift your left leg 12 inches higher, keeping your right leg stationary. Hold for 5 seconds. Put your legs together and slowly lower them to the floor. Repeat, raising your right leg. Do the entire sequence 5 times, working up to 10.

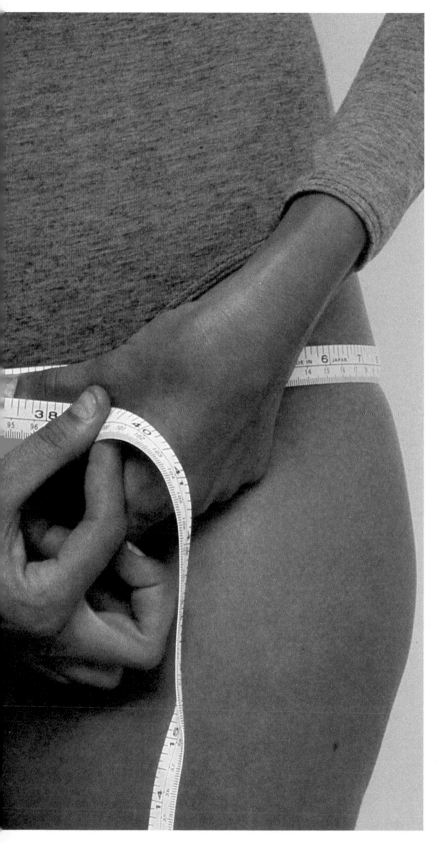

The best exercise for tightening your stomach and waist is swimming. It works every muscle in these areas. Concentrate on stretching your arms and legs. Reach as far as possible with every stroke.

Another good stomach and waist exercise is shown below. Lie on your right side, supporting your head with your hand. Lift your left leg slowly as high as you can. Only your leg should move. Your head, back and legs should remain in a straight line. Repeat this exercise 10 times with each leg, working up to 25.

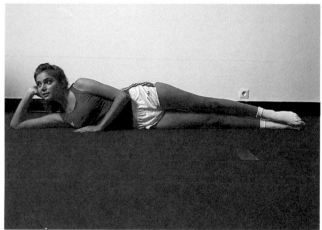

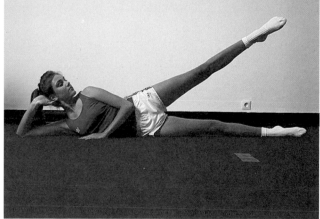

123

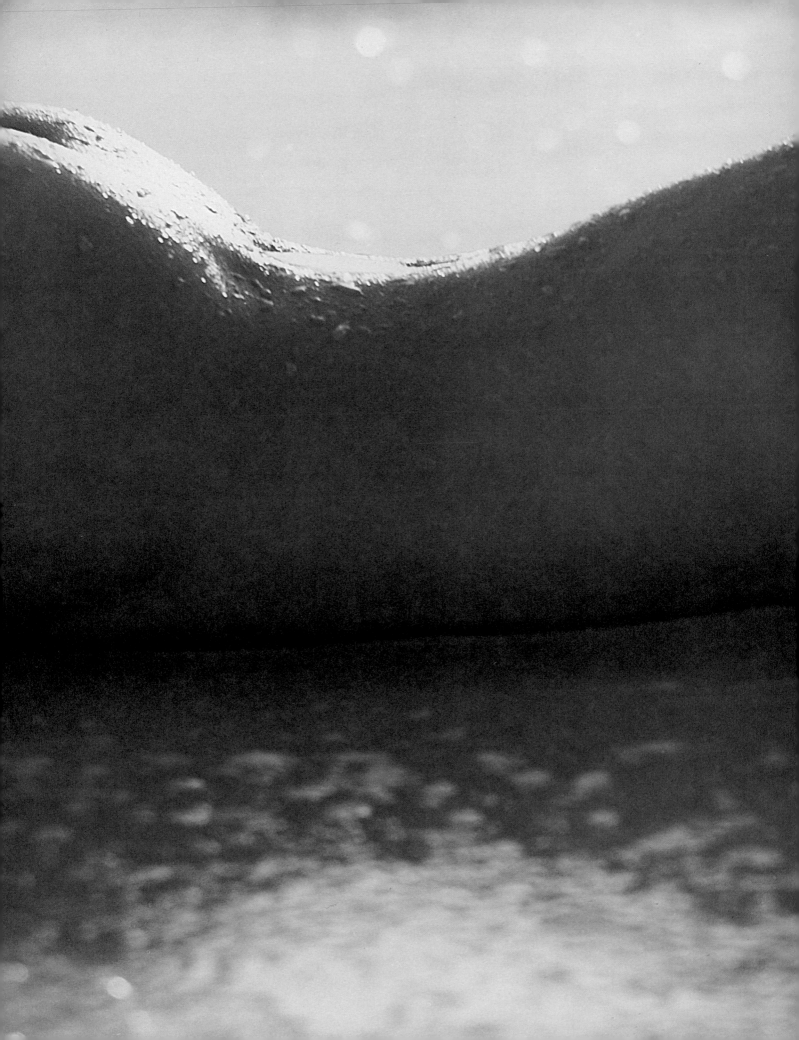

Back, Hips and Buttocks

Don't give your back the cold shoulder when it comes to skin care. If you turn your back on someone, it should at least be immaculate. A few minutes of daily care and an occasional special treatment will keep your back beautiful. Hips and buttocks will require more time. If yours aren't in good shape, only two things will help: exercise and diet. But it's worth the trouble to get these areas in shape. Then you can measure up to any critical glances. Even those behind your back.

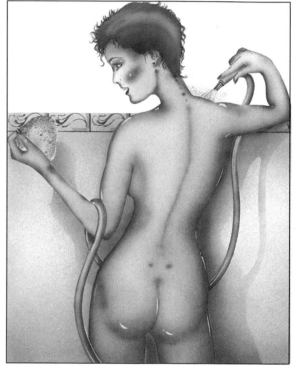

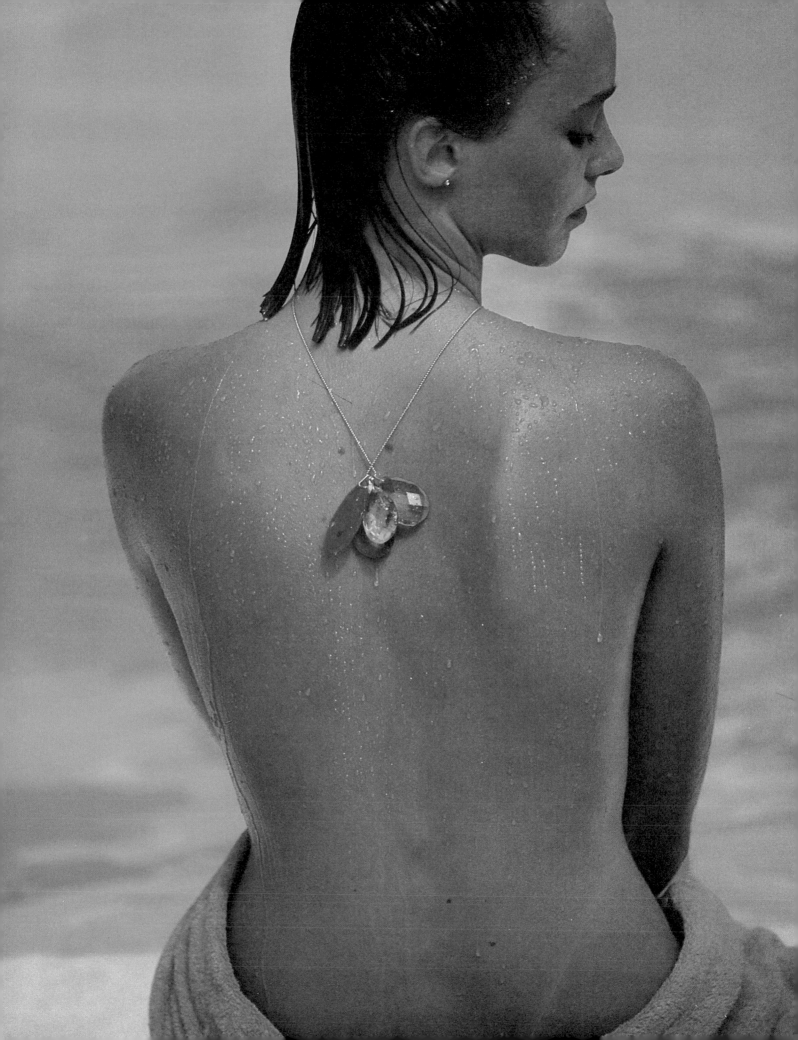

Back

The best exercise is the backstroke. You can also pamper your back at home or in the office with stretching exercises. They will relax your muscles and stimulate circulation.

Heat is the best treatment for backaches. Try soaking in a hot bath for 10 minutes. Then relax in bed under an electric blanket turned up high.

People seldom give their backs the treatment they deserve. Look at your back in the mirror from different angles. Is the skin oily or blemished? Bathing with a soap for oily skin will often take care

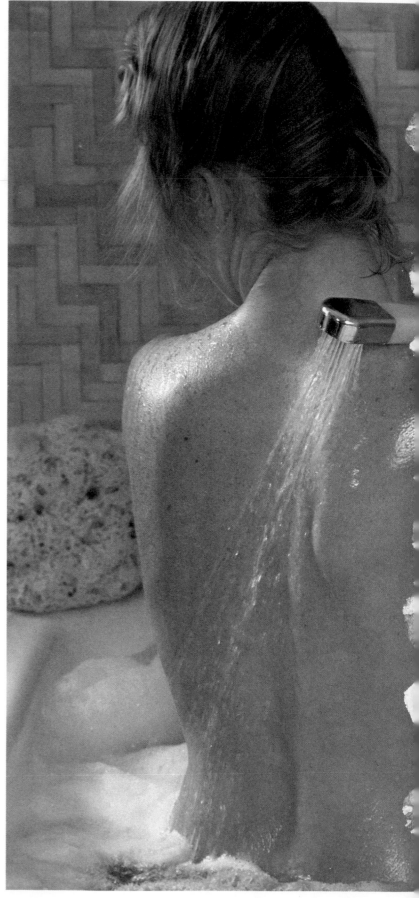

Vigorous massages with a brush, loofah sponge or shower-massage unit should be part of any beauty program. Massages improve circulation and make skin smooth and soft.

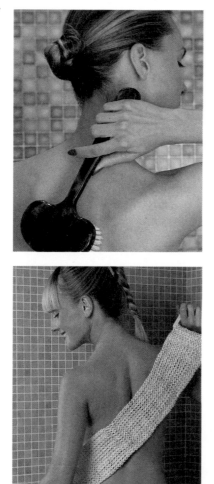

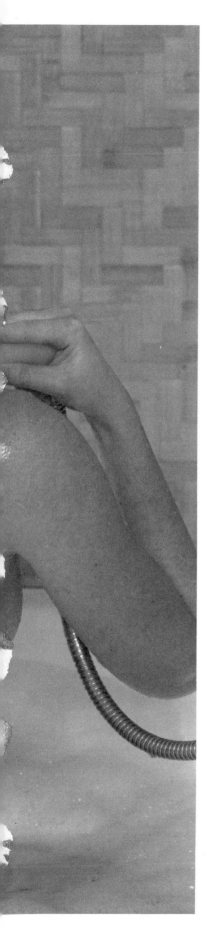

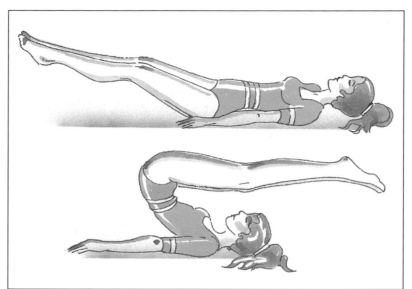

of this problem. You can also use acne preparations to clear up pimples. When you wear something cut low in the back, use an acne cream or lotion, then dust with antiseptic powder.

Even normal skin sometimes has problems. Here's a quick treatment you can use when your back is slightly blemished. Get circulation going with an exfoliant cream. If you don't have one, make a thick paste from salt and milk. Rub it vigorously into the skin.

Rinse off your skin thoroughly after this treatment. Cover with body lotion or moisturizing cream.

Exercise is an important aspect of back care. It doesn't matter whether your skin looks lovely if your muscles are tense and your back hurts.

Try this exercise for your back and the backs of your legs. Lie on the floor with your legs straight. Slowly raise your legs back over your head until your knees are above your nose. Keep the small of your back as close to the floor as possible. Hold your legs over your head 3 seconds, then slowly lower them to the floor. Repeat 5 times.

Hip and Buttock Exercises

Fat deposits on hips and buttocks are especially difficult to get rid of.

Don't expect quick results. Even if you do the four exercises shown on these facing pages regularly, you won't see major changes for several weeks.

Picture 1

Crouch on the floor and lean forward on your hands. Stretch one leg in back of you and lift it slowly. Tighten your buttocks and legs. Bounce your leg as high as you can 5 times. Slowly lower your leg, keeping it tensed. Relax and round your back. Switch legs and repeat. Do this sequence 10 times, working up to 25.

Picture 2

Lie on your back, arms out straight from the shoulders on the floor. Raise your legs straight up. Spread your legs, cross them, spread them again in quick, continuous movements. Inhale as you spread your legs, exhale as you cross them. Repeat 20 times, working up to 50. Lower your legs slowly and relax.

Picture 3

Lie on your back, arms out straight from the shoulders on the floor. Raise your legs straight up and cross them. Lower crossed legs slowly to one side, then raise them again. Lower your legs to the other side, then raise them. Inhale as you lower your legs, exhale as you raise them. Repeat 5 times, working up to 20.

These exercises help eliminate extra fat you get on buttocks and thighs when you spend 8 hours a day sitting in an office.

Picture 4

Get on your hands and knees. Your weight should be on your hands. Duck your head and pull your left leg forward. Try to touch your knee to your nose. Then extend your leg back and lift it as high as you can. Raise your head as you lift your leg. When your leg is as high as it can comfortably go, bounce it twice. This exercise should be done in one continuous motion, and you should keep your back straight. Repeat 10 times with each leg, working up to 20.

1

2

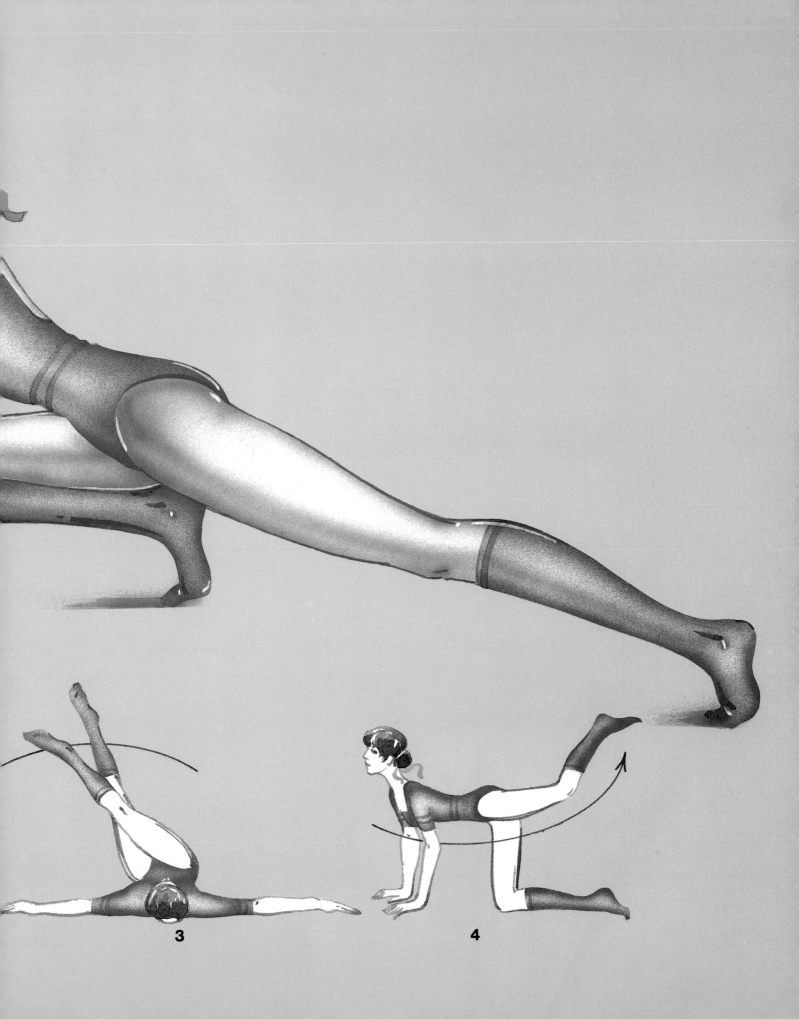

3

4

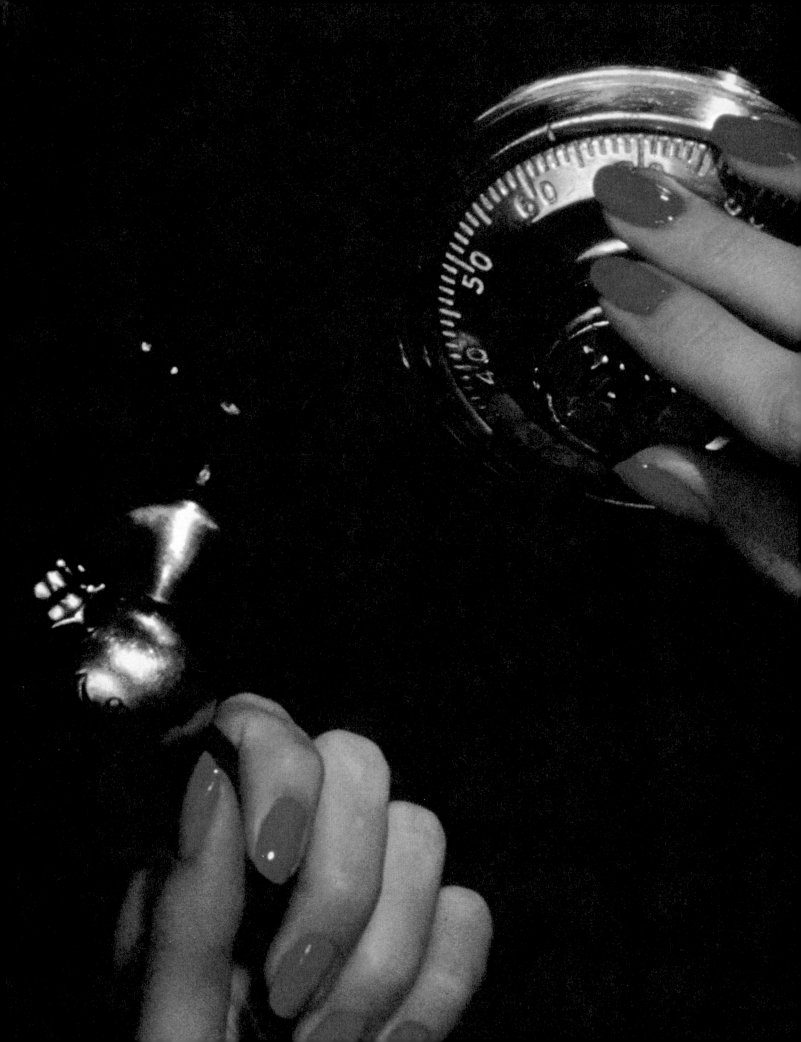

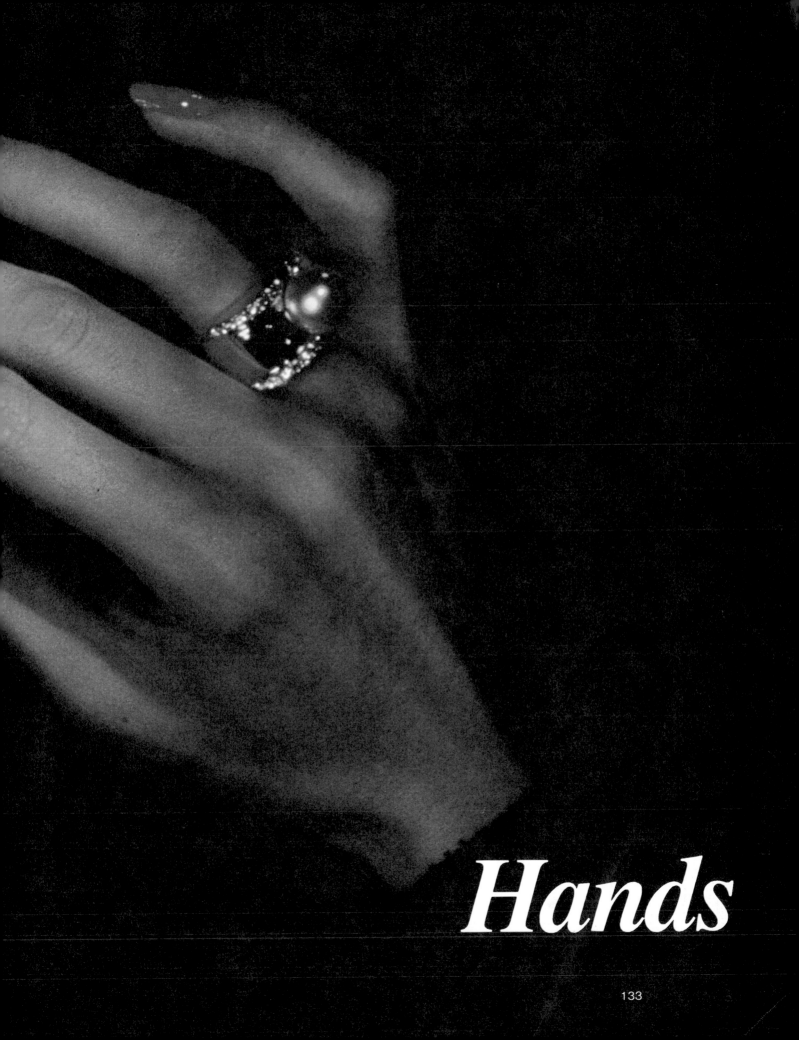

Hands

One way to draw attention to your hands is to wear large diamond rings. This isn't practical for most of us, however. We have to let our hands draw attention to themselves. Many people think hands, like eyes, tell a great deal about a person. So it's important to be sure your hands always look their best. On the following pages you will learn numerous ways to make your hands prettier. These include tips on manicures, exercise and massage. If you have a good hand-care program, you'll be glad when people watch your hands closely.

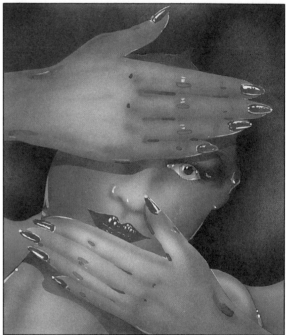

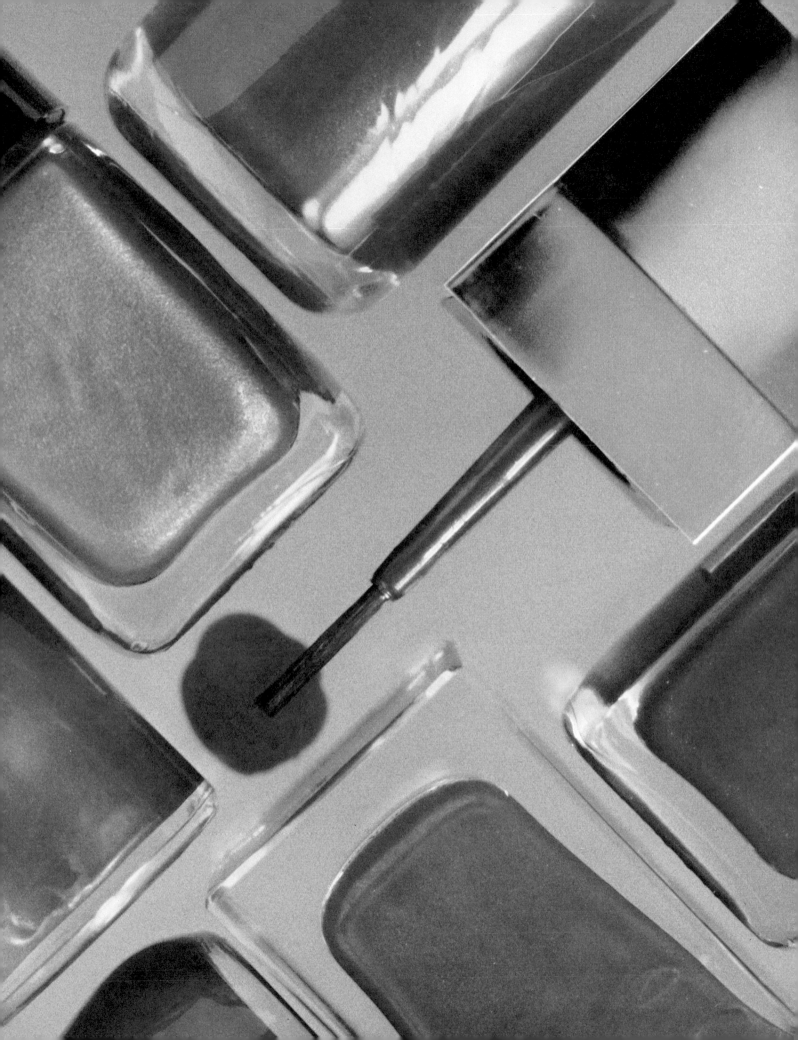

Manicure

You have to devote time to your hands once a week. They deserve it. They are constantly exposed to hot and cold air, wind, sun, dirt, soap and detergent.

Start your program by shaping your nails. Don't use scissors. You can cut too much off or make nails too lopsided. Don't use a metal file, either. It can heat up, causing nails to split. Use a diamond file or an emery board.

Gently file nails into an oval shape. Don't move the file forward and backward. File in one direction, from the outside toward the middle of the nail. This way the rim will be smooth.

Extremely long nails are neither fashionable nor practical. Well-cared-for hands have nails that project no more than a half inch beyond the fingertips.

After filing, wash fingertips

and pamper them by soaking them in warm, soapy water. This softens cuticles and loosens dirt. Treat discolored nails and fingers by squeezing lemon juice into the water.

Don't cut soft cuticles with scissors under any circumstances. It's better to apply cuticle remover, then gently push down cuticles and slide them off nails.

Cuticle removers are also available in the shape of a

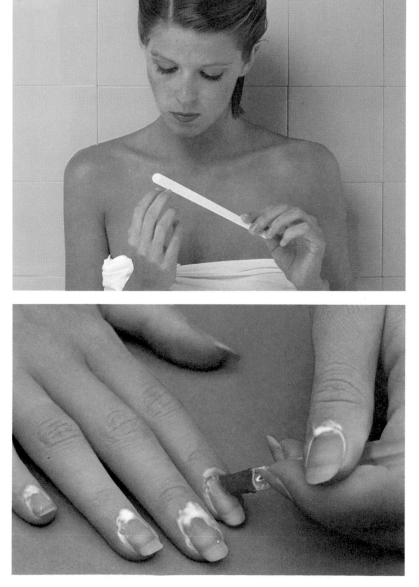

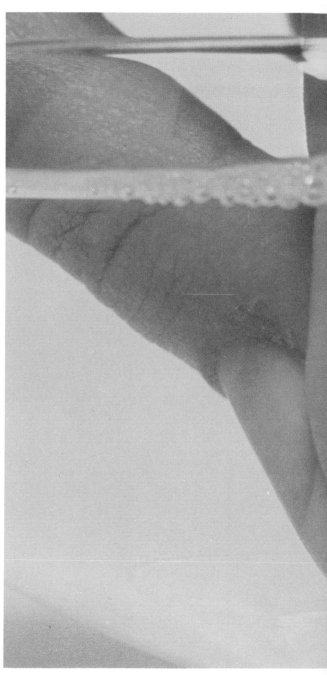

pencil. Remover is squeezed onto cuticles from one end of the pencil. Cuticles are pushed back and off nails with the other end.

You must be very gentle when dealing with your cuticles. They help prevent bacteria from attacking your nail tissue. If you damage your cuticles or use remover too frequently, you could develop an infection.

After using cuticle remover, wash your hands thoroughly. Then massage nail cream into the cuticle. The best time to do this is before going to bed, especially if you plan to wear nail polish. Polish doesn't adhere well to cream, so you shouldn't apply polish until the cream is completely dry.

To start your manicure, file nails, then wash fingertips thoroughly. Remove cuticles and massage nails with cream.

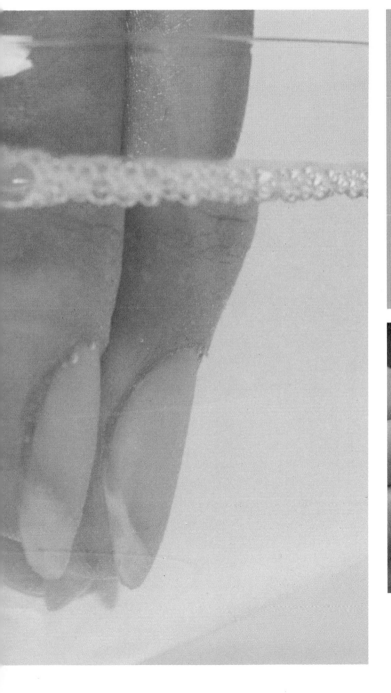

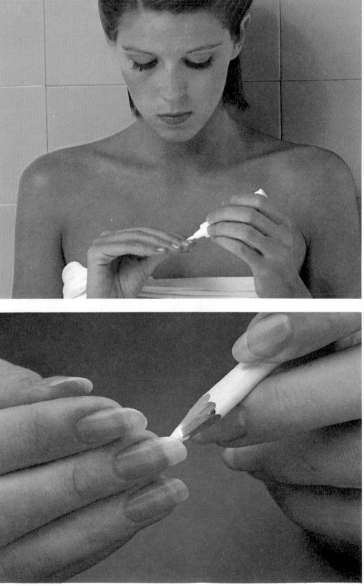

Polishing Techniques

Nails, like hair, are basically protein. They need natural oil to remain resilient. This oil is removed by soap, detergent and many nail polish removers.

To protect nails, choose polish remover carefully. It is much better to buy inexpensive nail polish than inexpensive remover. Be sure to buy a remover containing oil. Avoid removers containing acetone. They can make your nails brittle.

Polish can help your nails. It minimizes splits and breaks. Most polishes made by well-known companies are good quality. Price differences result from packaging. When you buy expensive polish you're usually paying more for the bottle, not the product.

Before polishing, be sure your nails are completely dry. Wait about an hour after bathing or washing dishes. This allows your nails, which absorb water, to shrink to normal size. If you polish wet nails, the polish will crack after several hours.

Put a base coat on the underside of the nail. This keeps dirt from accumulating there.

If you have soft nails, apply a strengthener. It prevents splits and breaks. Then apply a base coat. It smoothes uneven surfaces on your nails and prevents discoloration. After the base coat has dried, make a line with polish down the middle of your nail. Then fill in the sides.

You should dip the brush back in the bottle after each stroke. Wipe excess polish on the bottle neck. This is the only way you can get an even coat of polish.

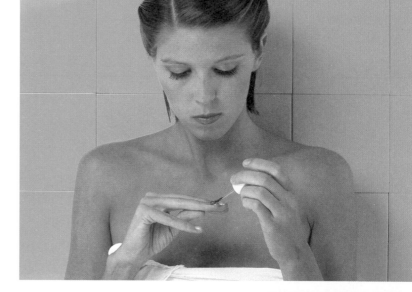

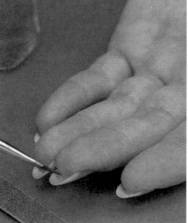

A thin base coat on the underside of nails prevents dirt from accumulating there. Dip the brush into the bottle before each stroke. Remove excess liquid by wiping brush on the bottle neck.

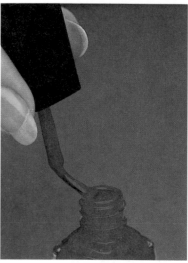

Apply a second coat of polish after the first has dried. If you get polish on the cuticle, remove it with a cotton swab or cotton ball soaked in polish remover.

After applying the last coat, wait at least 15 minutes before you handle anything. You may scratch your polish otherwise. If you're in a hurry, there is a spray that speeds drying. If you do not have the spray, put your hands under ice-cold water.

If polish chips off the end of your nail, dab a little polish on the bare spot. When this dries, give the entire nail another coat.

Never blow on your nails when they are drying. This can cause your polish to bubble and crack.

Make sure that the bottle cap and thread are free of polish. If you don't close the bottle tight, solvent in the polish evaporates, making polish thick and sticky. This can also happen if polish is stored in a warm place. Polish should remain thin and smooth for months if closed and stored properly.

To remove polish, put a little remover on a cotton ball. Run the cotton ball over the nail, wait a few seconds, then lightly rub the polish off.

Buffing brushes used before polish was invented are

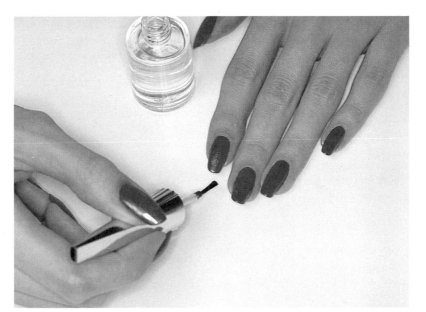

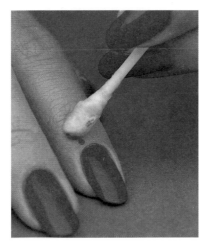

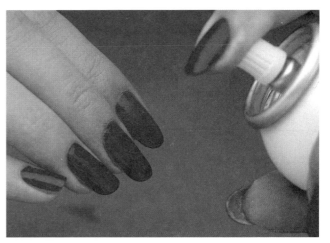

becoming fashionable again. Abrade nails slightly with the coarse side of the brush. This eliminates grooves. Buff nails with the other side of the brush. Nails will have a pretty, natural shine.

Apply a second coat of nail polish after the first has dried completely. If some polish misses the mark, remove it with a cotton swab soaked in polish remover. You can spray your polish to give it a hard finish.

Hand Exercises

Hands need to be exercised just like other parts of your body. Regular workouts strengthen muscles, promote agility and improve the shape of your hands.

Picture 1
Press your palms and fingertips together tightly. Move fingertips back and forth, bending your fingers as far as you can.

Picture 2
Press your hands together. Open them until only the palms of your hands remain touching. Bend your fingers back as far as you can.

Pictures 3 and 4
Straighten your fingers. Hold your hands still and swing your thumbs to the right 10 times, to the left 10 times and then tightly against your palms. Hold the thumbs against your palms for 5 seconds.

You should also massage your hands. Grab a finger of one hand with the thumb, index finger and second finger of the other. Massage from fingertip to wrist. Do this with each finger and the thumb on each hand. Put moisturizing cream or lotion on your hands before starting this massage.

Moisturizers are an important part of hand care. You should apply them each time you wash your hands. Never put your hands in dishwater unless you have on rubber gloves.

You can make your hands prettier with exercise, massage and regular manicures.

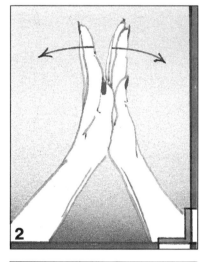

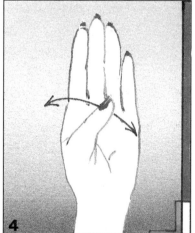

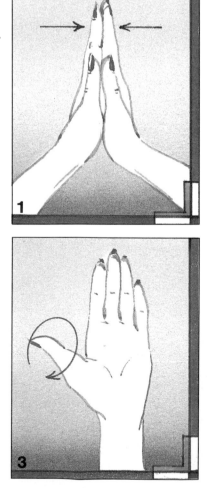

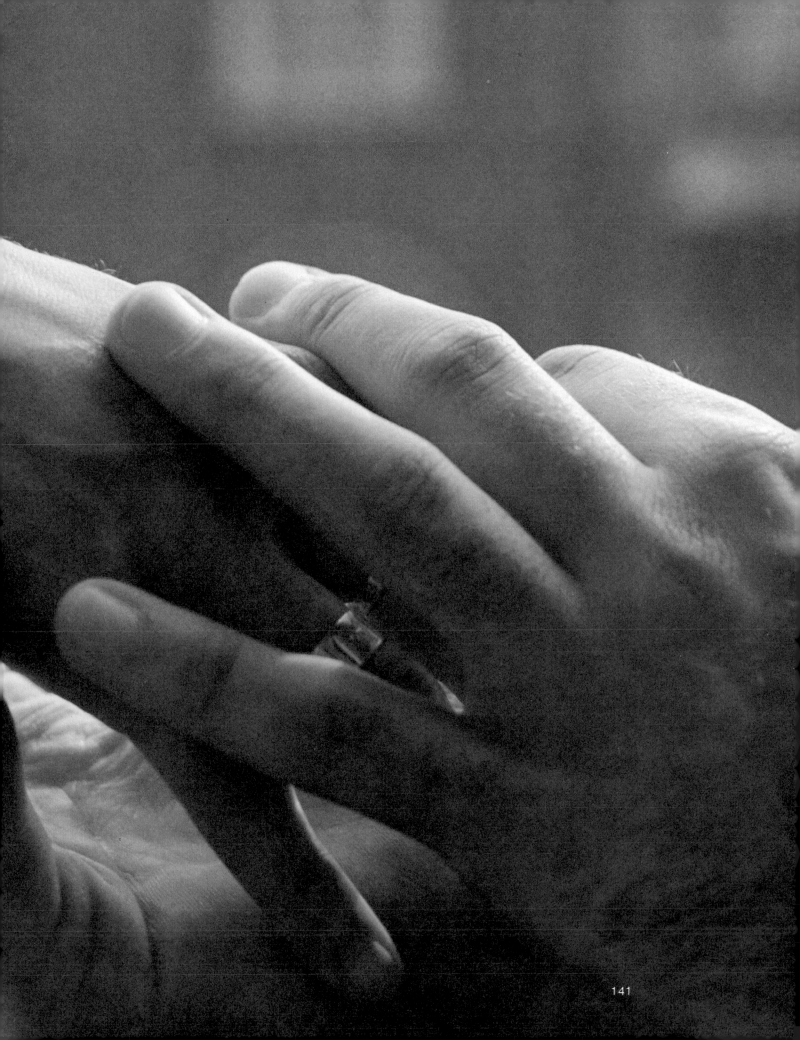

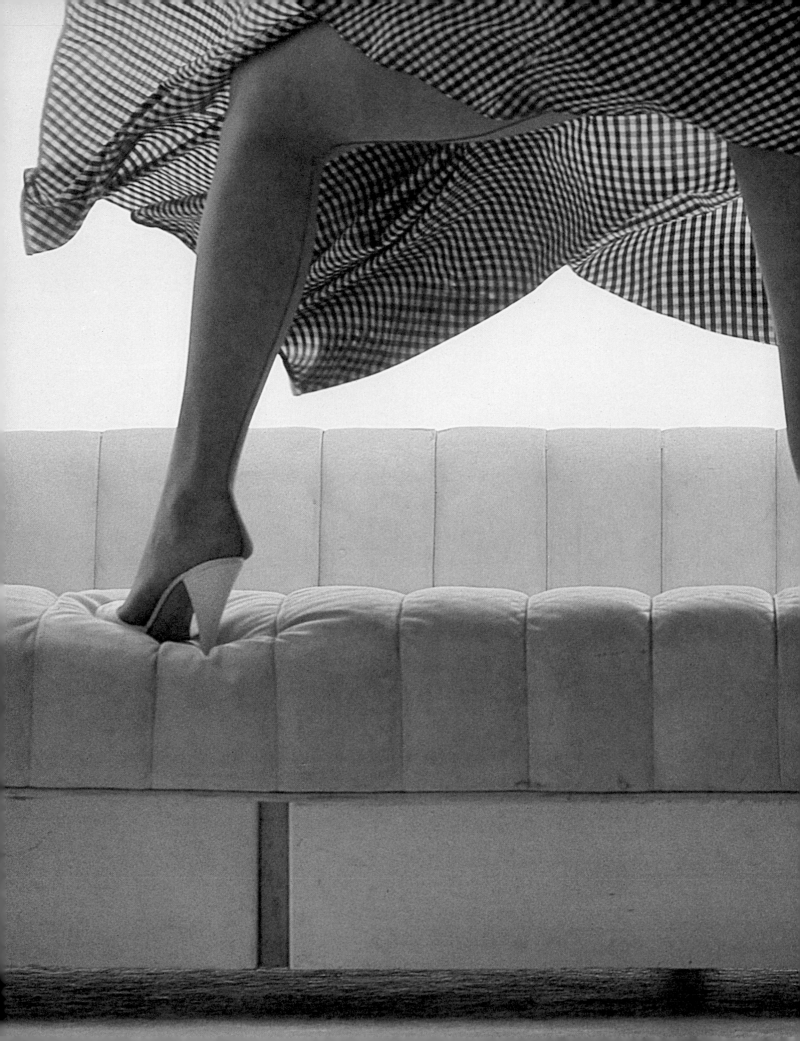

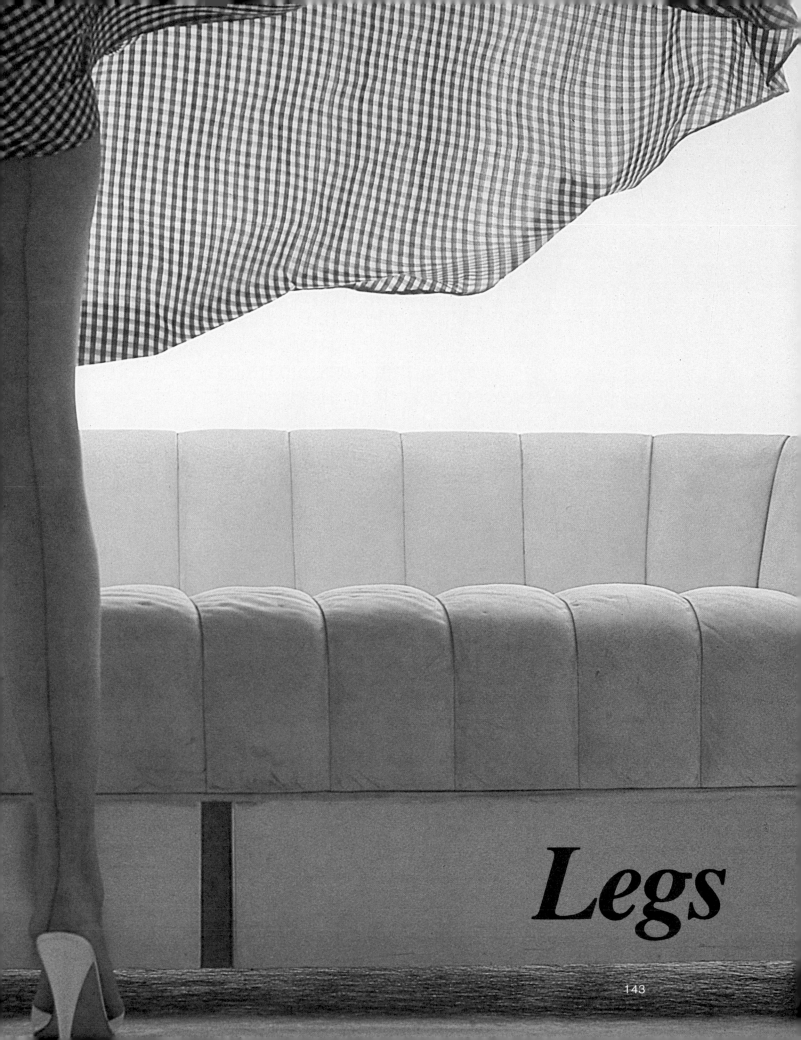

Legs

You step lightly from the house on pretty legs in the morning and trudge home on sore, tired legs in the evening. Legs can quickly become your major beauty problem. Heat makes them swell. Tight boots make them ache. Standing for hours causes them to develop varicose veins. Don't let the situation get out of hand. Stand firm in your resolve to give leg care high priority.

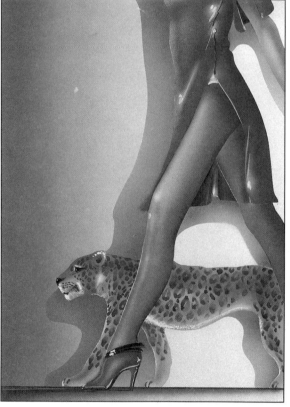

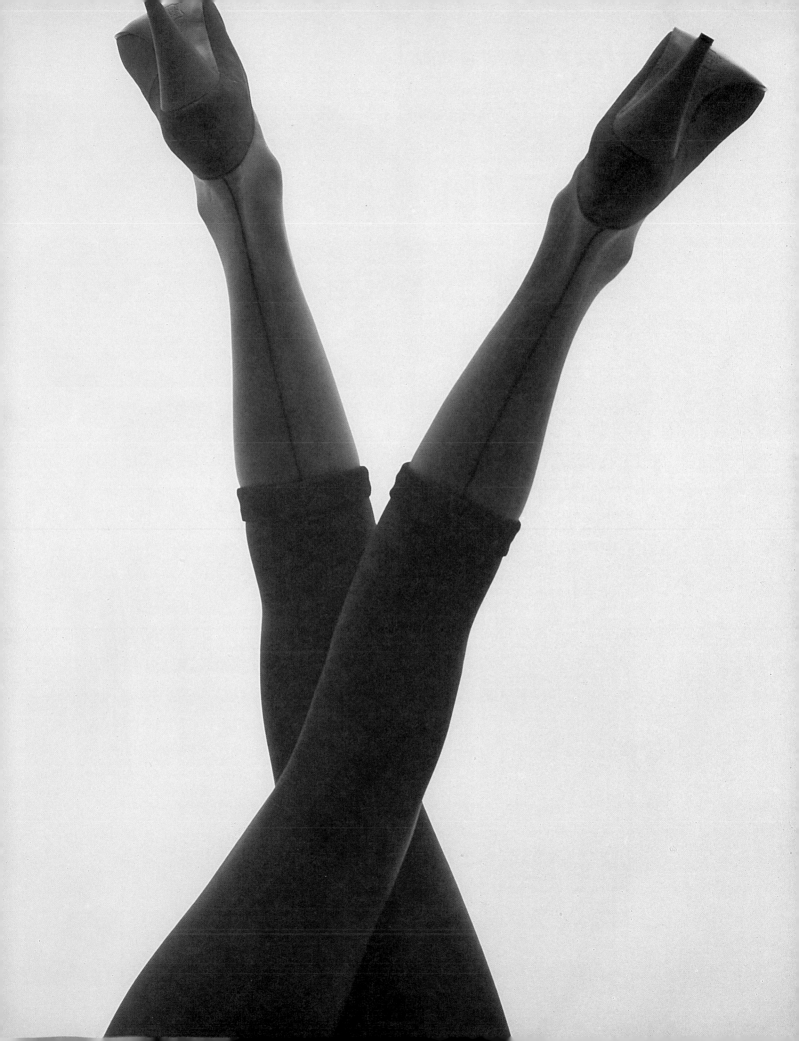

Hair Removal

You can easily remove unwanted hair yourself. The principal hair-removal methods are creams, lotions, wax, shaving and electrolysis.

Creams and Lotions—These hair removers, called *depilatories,* contain a chemical compound that dissolves hair. It takes about 10 days for hair to grow out.

You can use either creams or lotions. Both give similar results. Test for allergic reaction beforehand. Sensitive skin may become red and irritated.

Depilatories formulated for the face also work well in the pubic area. Use the mildest cream or lotion available. It will keep your bikini line soft and smooth.

Before using cream or lotion hair remover, put a little on the inside of your arm. Leave it for 10 minutes to test for allergic reaction.

Creams and lotions have two major disadvantages. They are expensive and they take time—at least 20 minutes.

Shaving—This method is more effective if you use an electric shaver. Buy one with a rotating head that will adjust to the shape of your legs and underarms.

An electric shaver works best when skin is free of oil. Plan to shave every 2 to 3 days.

Using wax to remove hair requires some skill. Have your cosmetologist show you the proper technique. You can burn yourself severely if you don't use wax carefully.

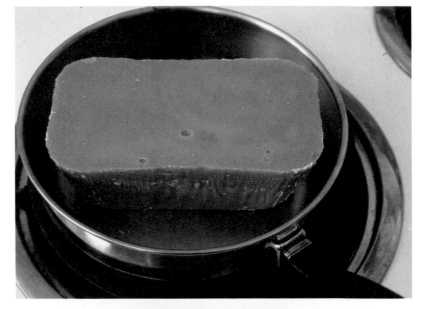

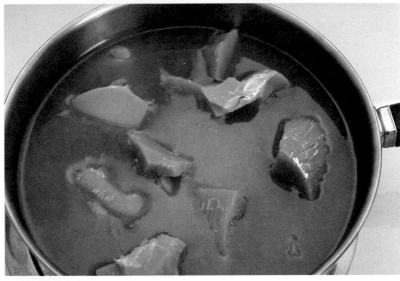

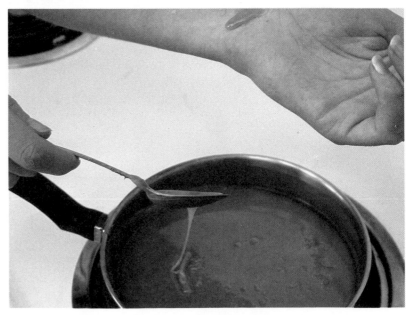

If you use a razor, buy one with a curved head. You are less likely to cut yourself. Be sure blades are new and clean. Soap your legs and underarms well before you start shaving.

Waxing—This is a long-term solution to hair growth. Skin will remain smooth for as long as 4 weeks. You can use wax strips or tablets. You press ready-to-use strips directly on the hair. Leave the strip in place for the recommended time. Then peel off the strip, moving against the direction of the hair growth.

You melt wax tablets and apply them warm. Doing this correctly requires practice. *You can burn yourself severely,* so let an experienced cosmetologist show you the proper technique.

Electrolysis—Hair doesn't grow back after electrolysis, which destroys hair follicles.

The person performing this procedure must treat each follicle individually, so this hair-removal technique is very expensive and time-consuming. It can also be somewhat painful.

Electrolysis should be done only by a highly trained professional. Be sure to check the credentials of the person you're considering.

Moisten your legs before applying a depilatory. This enables the cream or lotion to work faster. Wipe off the depilatory and loosened hair with a spatula or rough washcloth. Then rinse legs well and apply moisturizing cream.

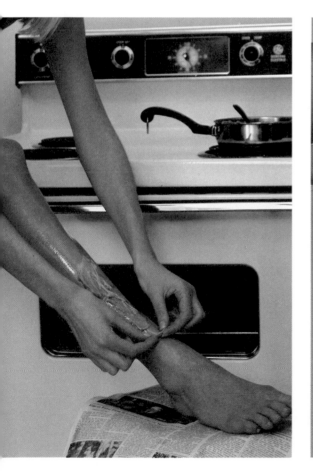

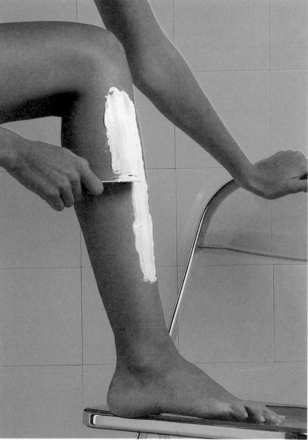

Leg Care

Begin your leg-care program with daily brushing and massage. Brush with either a loofah sponge or body brush. The best time to massage is during your shower. Begin at the ankles and move upward with circular motions to the buttocks.

Also knead your thighs. Start at the knees and work upward, using both hands. Don't grab too much skin or pinch too hard. Grab the skin with your thumb and index finger, pull for a second, then let go.

When you finish your massage, rinse off in cold water.

If you notice marks on your calf or in the bend of your knee that look like red or blue spiders, see a dermatologist. In most cases these veins can be eliminated by cauterization or injections.

You can help prevent these veins by avoiding tight boots and shoes with spike heels. Elevating your feet whenever possible is also beneficial.

Many women consider dimples and ripples, popularly known as *cellulite,* a special beauty problem, but it isn't. Each individual has specific areas where fat becomes concentrated. In women, these usually include the thighs and buttocks. The skin in these areas develops an orange-peel look. However, cellulite is not a medical term. It is nothing more than normal fatty tissue.

Here's a quick exercise to relax your legs. Lean on the back of a chair and bend your right leg. Raise up on the toes of your left foot. Hold 5 seconds, then slowly lower foot to the floor. Repeat, bending your left leg, and raising up on the toes of your right foot. Do this 5 times.

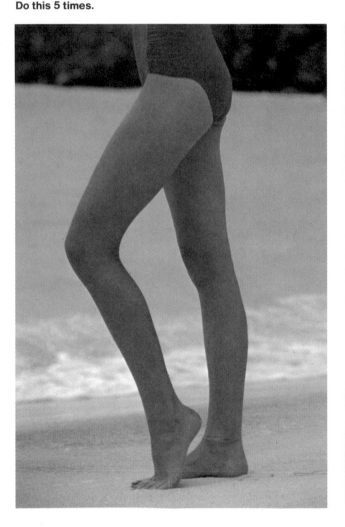

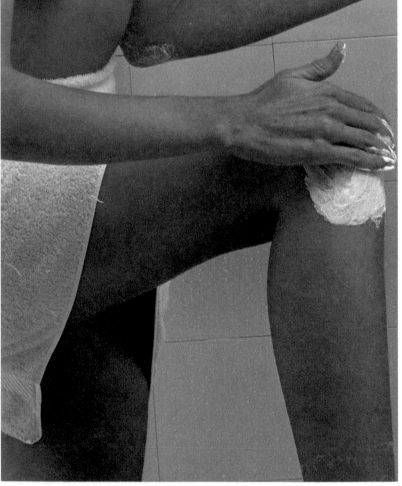

148

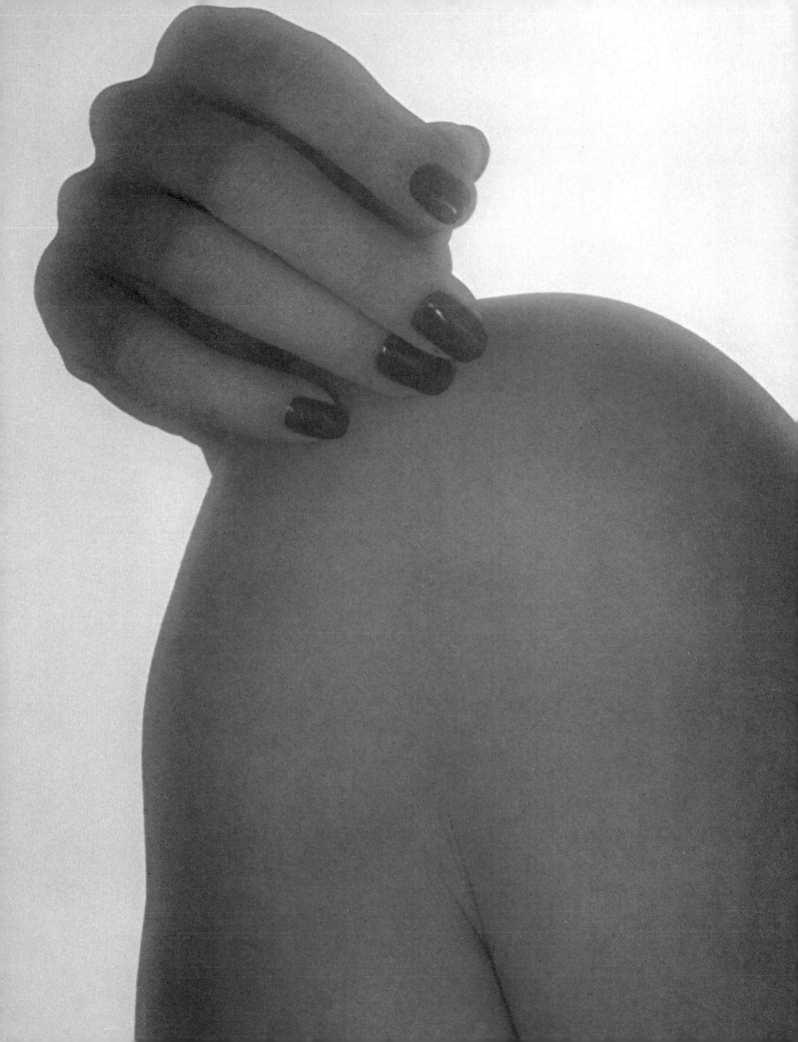

Varicose Veins

Varicose veins are unsightly. Do your best to prevent them. A predisposition to varicose veins is hereditary, so if anyone in your family has developed them, you should be especially diligent.

If varicose veins spread quickly or become painful, see a physician. Your doctor can determine whether major veins or arteries are involved. If they are, varicose veins could be indicative of a blockage or

doctor who specializes in varicose vein treatment.

Varicose veins require surgery only in serious cases. Your doctor may recommend it if varicose veins hurt or repeatedly become inflamed.

The best thing to do is prevent the development of these veins.

Wear support stockings and elevate your legs whenever possible.

Avoid clothes that restrict

circulation. These include tight pants and girdles, and knee socks.

Stimulate your circulation every way you can. Walk and exercise daily.

If you are taking oral contraceptives, discuss trying another form of birth control with your physician. Women with a family history of diseases involving the blood vessels should seriously consider another form of birth control.

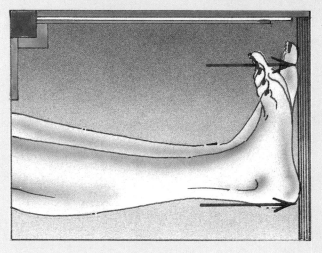 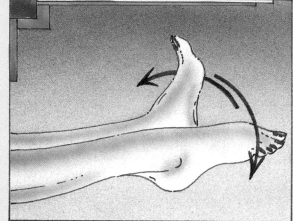

blood clot that should be treated immediately.

If you have only a few varicose veins, a doctor can cauterize them. This procedure involves removing blood from the veins and filling them with a *sclerosing agent,* which seals off the veins. The procedure is harmless and not painful. Numerous injections will be necessary, however. Insurance companies sometimes cover treatment costs. Choose a

To help prevent varicose veins, elevate your legs whenever you can. Flexing your feet in the manner shown in the illustrations above can also be beneficial.

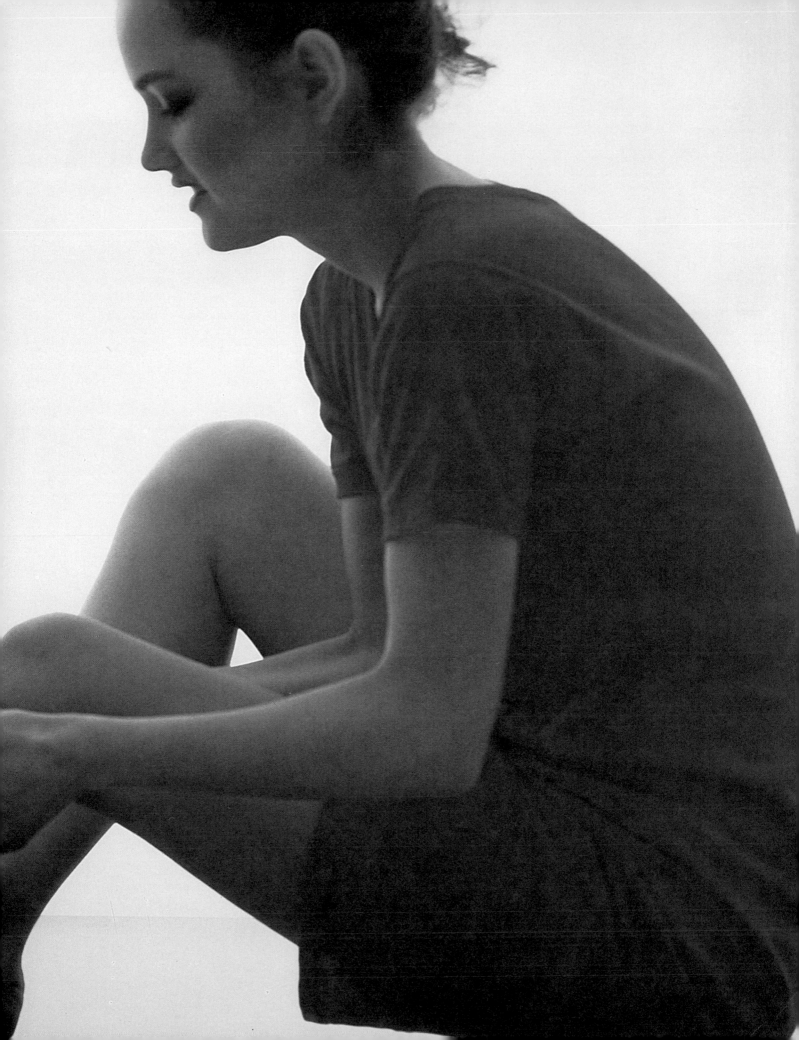

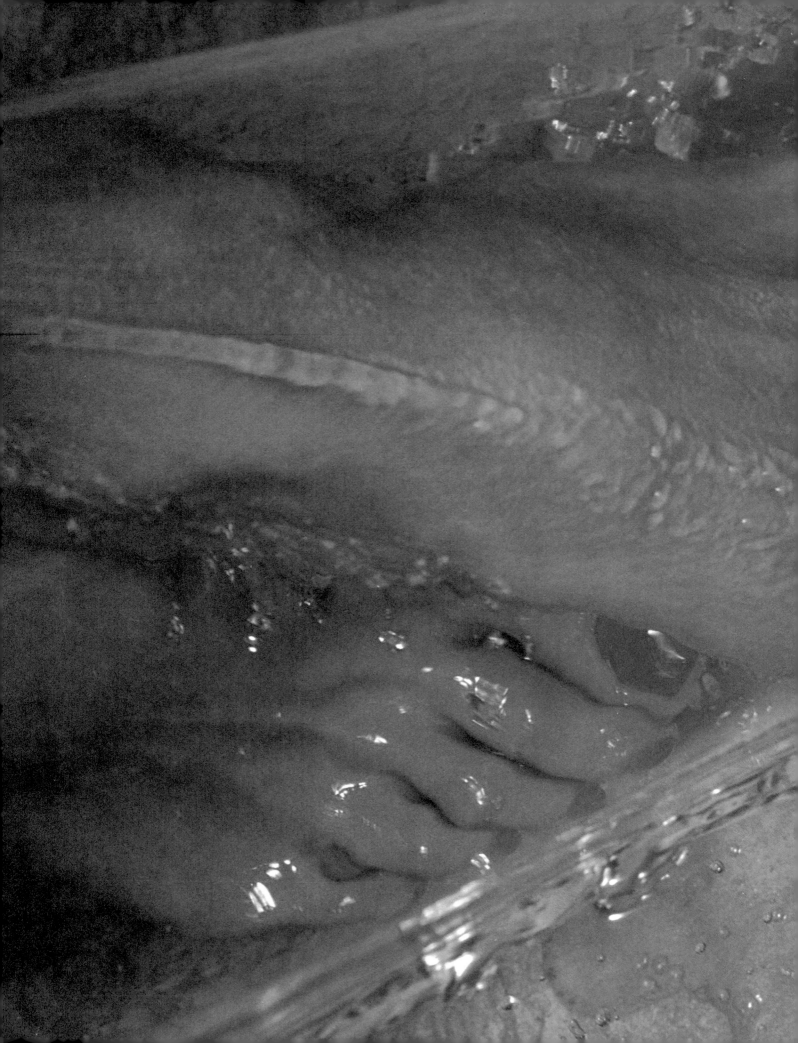

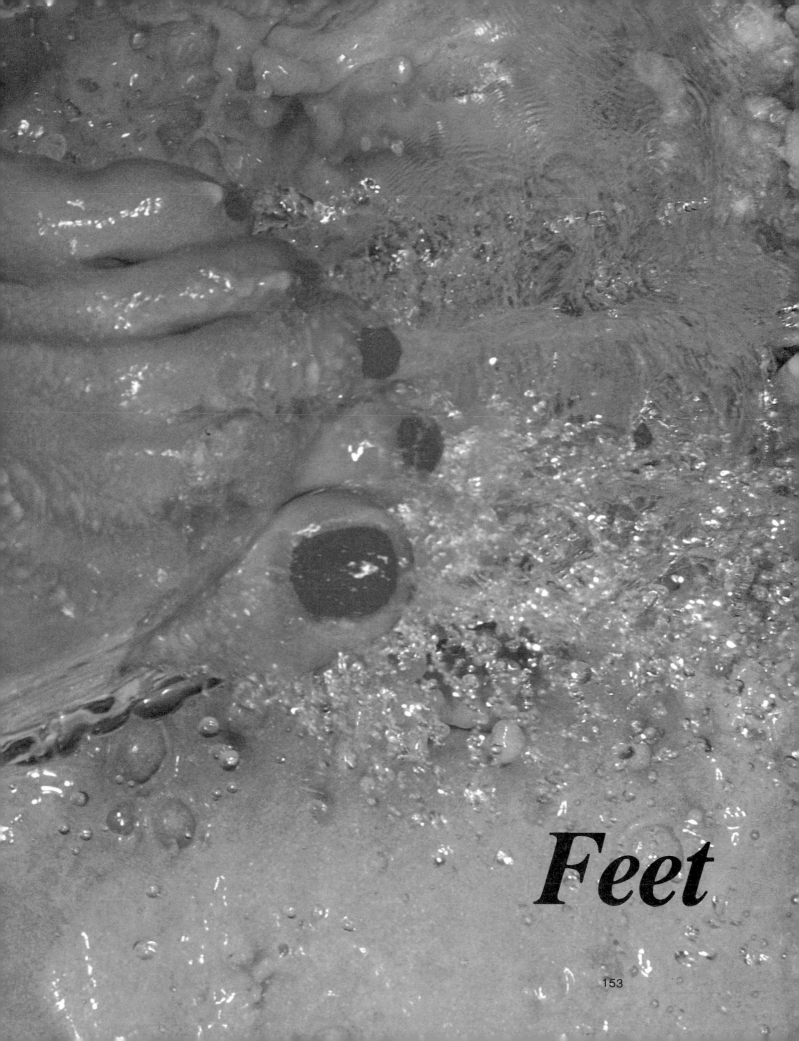

Feet

Do you pay attention to your feet only when they hurt? Remember that feet have their own beauty. Think about a delicate foot whose pretty, polished nails shimmer through a sheer stocking. Wouldn't you like your feet to look like that? All your feet need to be more attractive is proper care. This should take 2 minutes every day and a half hour once a week. The effort is worth it. Don't you want to be prepared in case someone should throw himself at your feet?

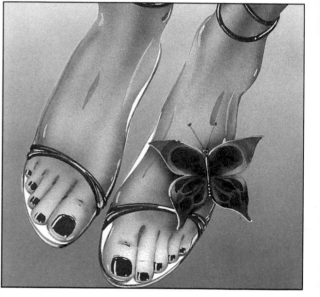

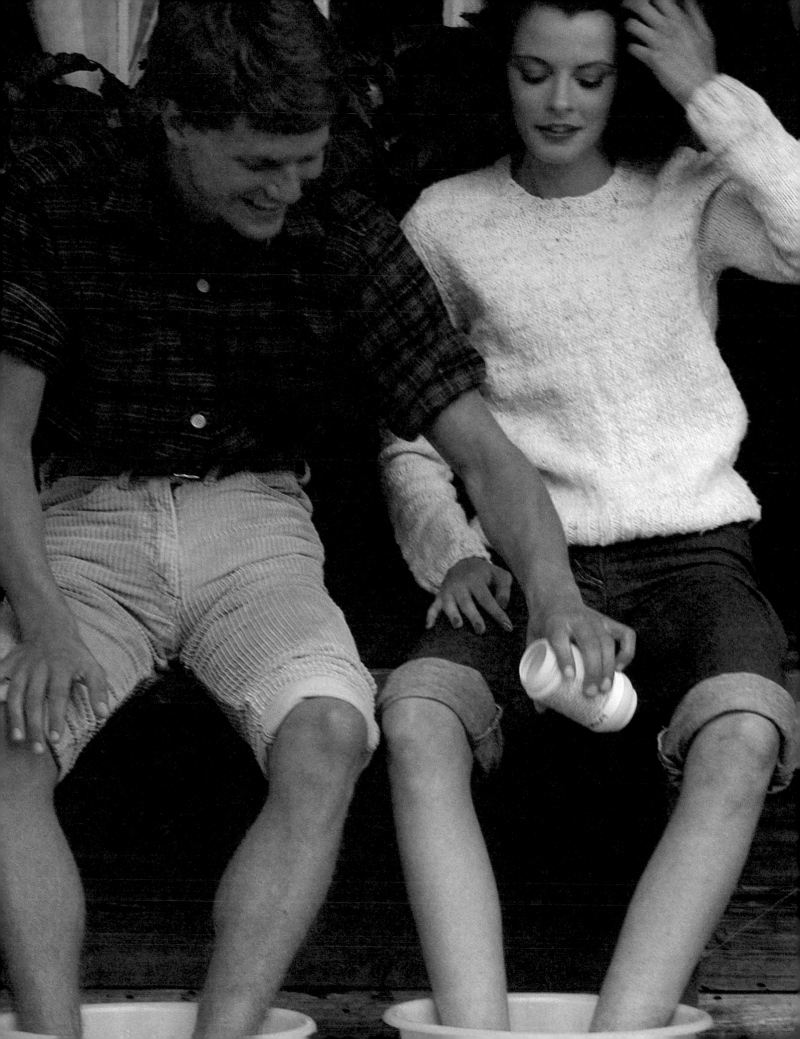

Pedicure

Begin by soaking your feet in lukewarm water for approximately 5 minutes. This softens toenails and the thick skin on the balls and heels of your feet and on your toes. Trim your toenails with nail clippers or nail scissors. Toenails should be short and clipped in a straight line across the top. Oval-shaped toenails can become painfully ingrown on the sides.

Afterward, smooth nails with a file so they can't snag stockings. Rub callouses with a pumice stone. Callous files can also be used, but they work better on dry skin. Handle files carefully. You can scrape off too much skin.

Put everything you need within easy reach before starting your foot treatment.

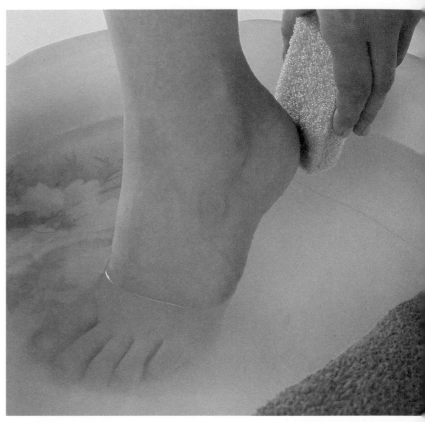

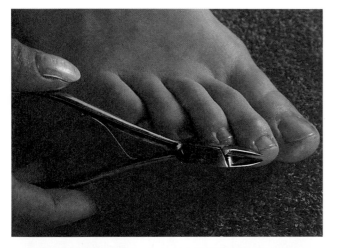

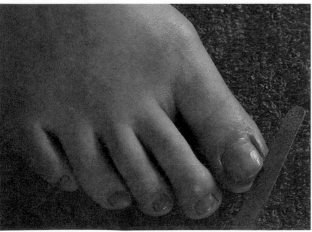

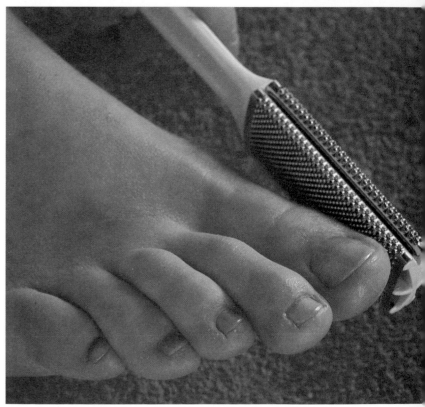

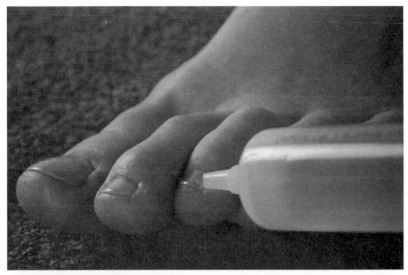

Special lotions are also available that remove rough, dry skin.

Try one or a combination of these methods and see which works best for you.

Be sure to use cuticle remover on each toenail. Cuticles should be pushed back and off the nail. Toenails should then be scrubbed with a nail brush to eliminate all unwanted skin particles.

The nails are now ready for polish. Put cotton balls or tiny foam rubber wedges between the toes. This will enable you to reach each nail easily and will minimize smudging.

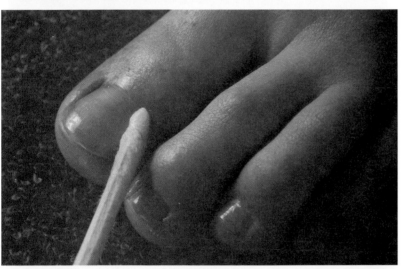

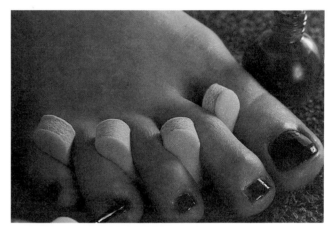

When polish has dried completely, put moisturizing cream or body lotion on your feet. This refreshes and protects your skin.

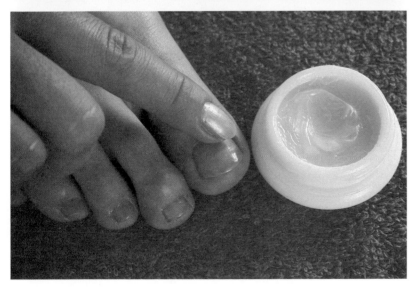

Tips for Pretty, Healthy Feet

Your feet work hard every day. You can keep them fit by giving them special treatment occasionally.

A pressure massage wakes up swollen, tired feet. Take each toe between your thumb and index finger and apply strong pressure with the thumb on three spots: the cuticle area, behind the toe joint and at the base of the toe.

Then massage the top and bottom of each foot. Start with the spaces between the toes and move down to the instep. Then start at the heel and move along the instep to the ball of the foot

and the Achilles' tendon. Next, go slowly up the ankle. Massage each foot for 3 minutes, then elevate your legs for 10 minutes.

Exercise also helps keep your feet in shape. Put the sole of your foot on a small, hard ball and move it in all directions.

If you've been on your feet all day, a footbath with bath salts can be very therapeutic. If you use lukewarm water, leave your feet in about 10 minutes. It's better to alternate warm and cold water. Add salt to the warm water and soak feet about

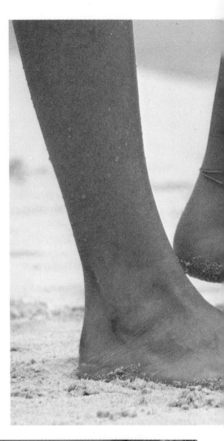

Massage, exercise and bright nail polish make your feet more attractive.

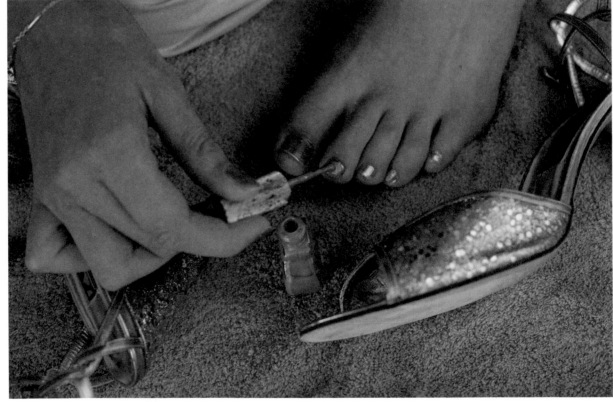

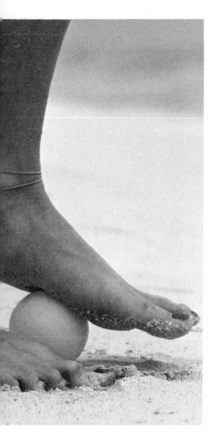

5 minutes. Move feet to the cold water and soak them for 3 minutes. Be sure to end the footbath with your feet in cold water.

If your feet hurt, you may be wearing shoes that are slightly too small or too narrow. The most healthful shoes for your feet are sandals. They allow your feet to breathe and also show them off very well. When you wear sandals, use extra-special nail polish. Try an extraordinary color, such as lilac or hot pink. Or use polish with a gold shimmer.

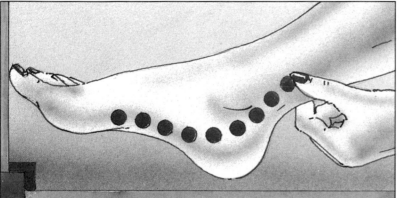

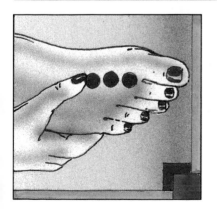

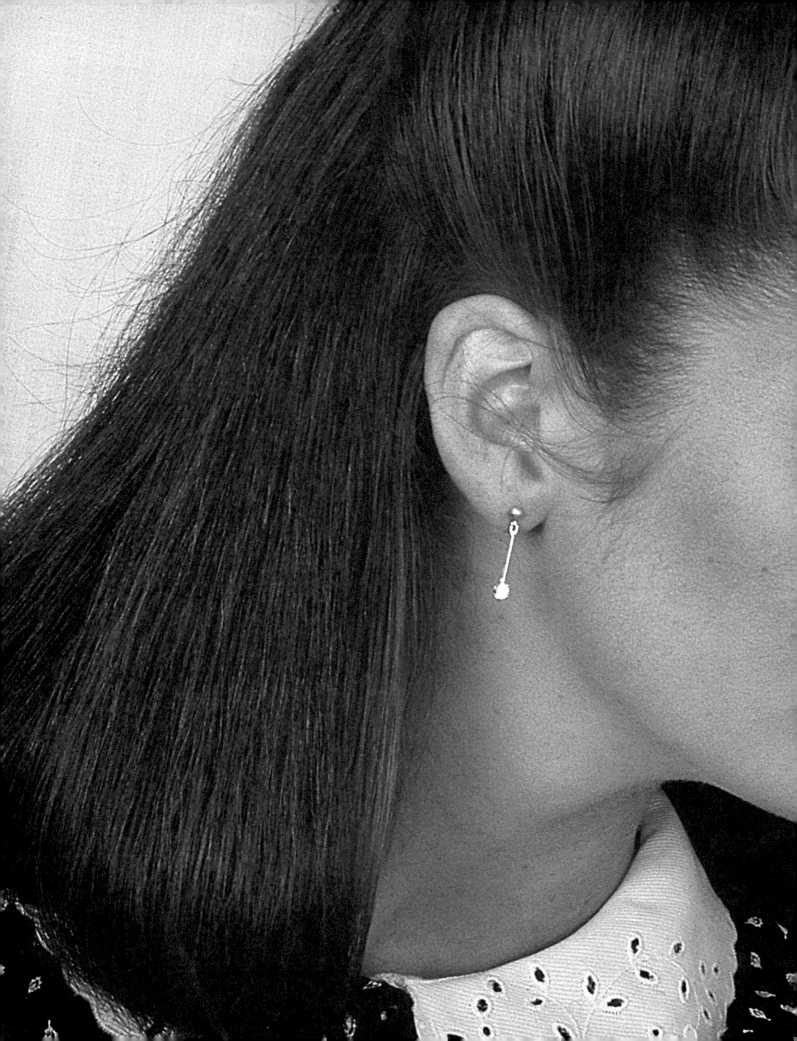

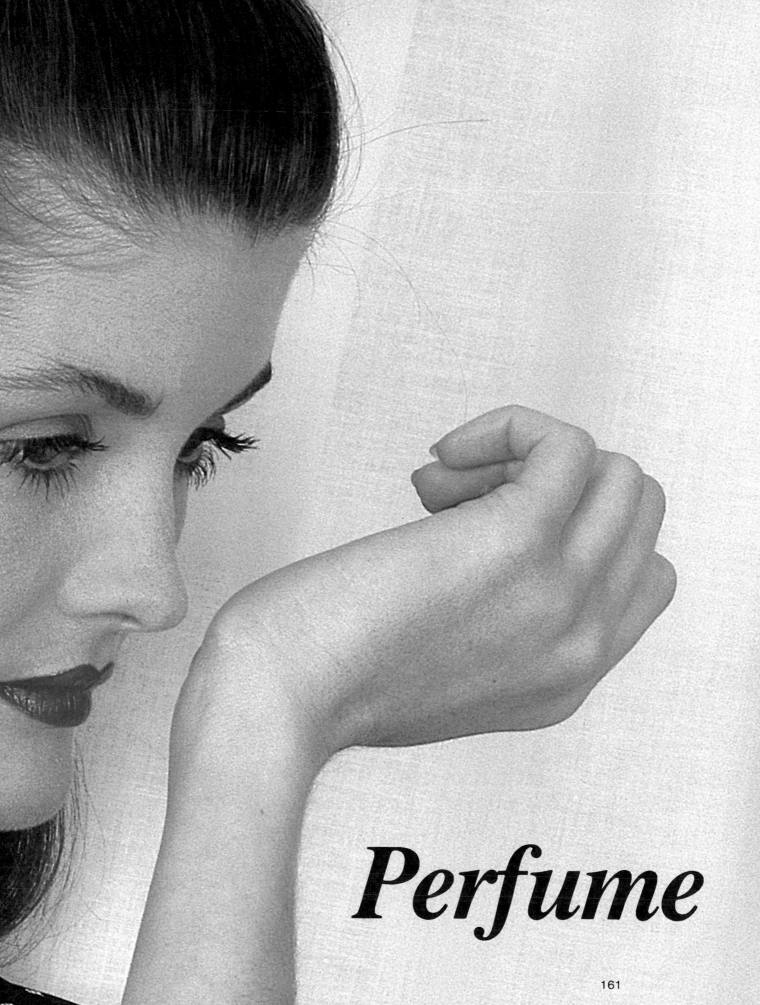

Perfume

Perfume is a luxury. We spoil ourselves with it. It is also a cunning way of communicating. We can use it to tell others how we feel and what we have planned. Naturally, this works only if you have a fitting scent for every occasion. For official gatherings, you need an elegant scent. It will be noticed by everyone without being obtrusive. For romantic excursions, you need a quiet, dreamy scent that will slowly permeate the senses of your companion. For work 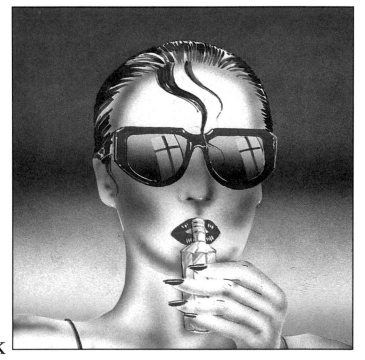 and everyday outings, you need a clean, fresh scent. So join the fragrance game. Make it a habit to wear a different perfume with jeans than with a silk dress.

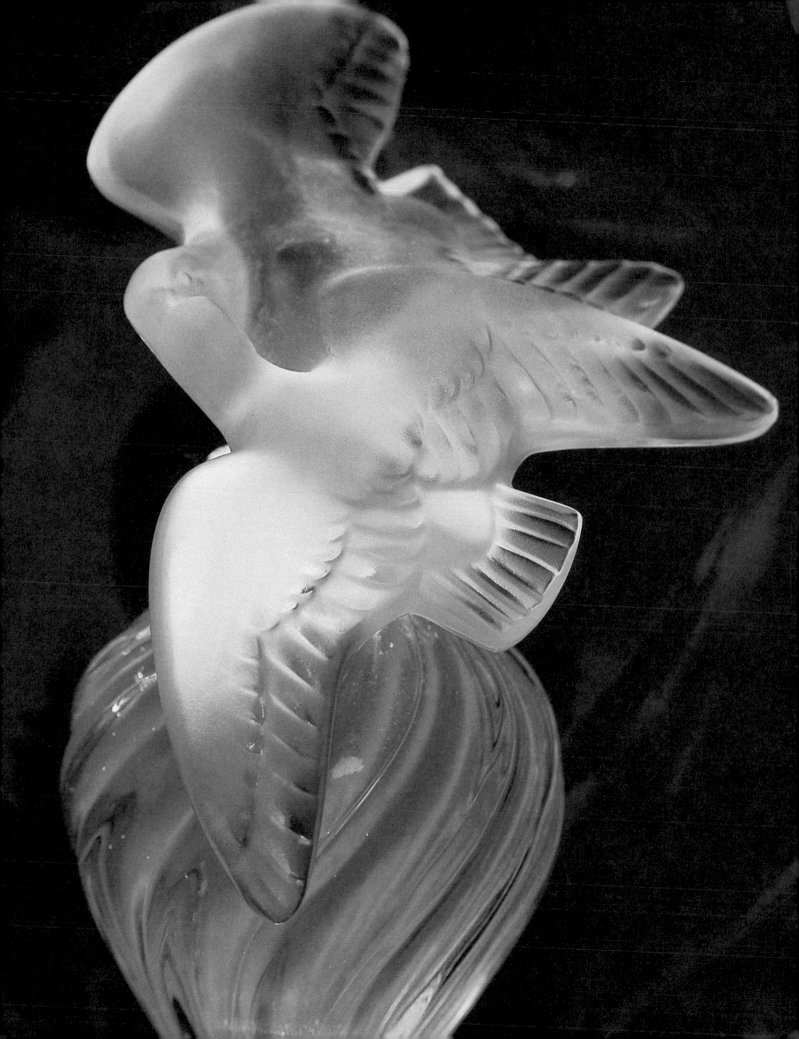

Finding the Right Fragrance

The scent of your perfume can change from one minute to the next. That's because the ingredients do not evaporate at the same rate. Some develop their scent immediately. Others need hours.

Perfume is like a musical composition. What you detect just after applying it are the opening notes of the scent. Perfume manufacturers call these *top notes*. They arouse interest and draw attention

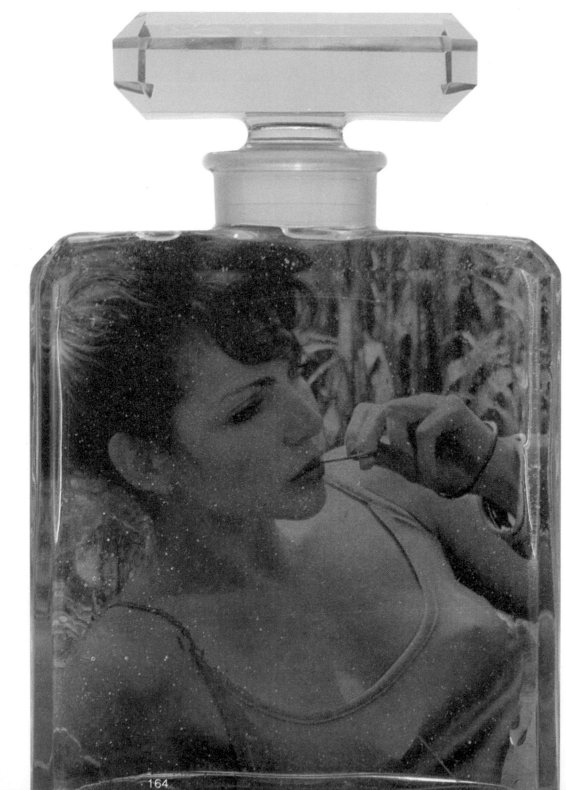

with their charm.

The body of the scent, called the *middle note,* is more hearty and long-lasting. It unfolds slowly, over 4 to 5 hours, and gives the perfume its distinctive character. The *end note* or *base note* of the scent is quiet and soft. It is the scent that lingers on your skin and clothing.

Eau de cologne is different. The fresh, fleeting opening notes set the tone for the scent, so they are less intense than the opening notes of perfume. Another difference is that perfume is approximately 35% scent concentrate and eau de cologne is 3 to 8%.

Between perfume and eau de cologne are scented waters such as eau de toilette and day perfumes. Each brand has a different proportion of scent concentrate. Some contain as much concentrate as perfume. Others contain as much as eau de cologne. All have a more refreshing effect on skin than perfume.

You need time to buy perfume. A person's sense of smell tires quickly. Before long, you can't differentiate one perfume from another. Never sample more than three scents at one time. And never try more than two on yourself, one on each wrist.

One helpful hint is to bring along scent strips. You can make them from coffee filters, which are absorbent and have no scent of their own. Cut the filters into strips and let the salesperson spray a fragrance on each. Over the hours you can compare how different fragrances develop.

Use this only to make your initial selection. Your final choice must depend on how each scent develops on your skin.

Once you've narrowed the field to three or four perfumes, ask the salesperson for a sample of each. Perfume manufacturers send samples to be given to customers so they can become familiar with different scents.

If the store doesn't carry samples, return in the morning—without using perfume—and use a tester to spray yourself. Then see how the scent changes throughout the day. You will have to return to the store several times to try the perfumes you're interested in, but it's worth the trouble. Wearing each perfume for an entire day will give you an excellent idea of what each scent is like.

Don't throw away empty perfume bottles. Leave them open in your closet so your clothing will smell nice, too.

If you can't decide between two perfumes, buy both. Above all, perfumes are a matter of mood. Today you may want a floral scent, tomorrow an exotic one. But if you like to change fragrances frequently, remember that perfume adheres to clothing.

When buying perfume, remember that different perfumes work best in different seasons. In summer, a perfume's fragrance is more intense and doesn't last as long. Light, flowery scents you can spray on several times a day are recommended.

In the winter, heavy, exotic perfumes work best. They exude warmth on cold nights.

Perfume is also affected by geography. In humid places, perfume is stronger but evaporates faster. Delicate, fresh scents are needed.

If you are living in or visiting a coastal area, remember that sea air overpowers many perfumes. Try spicy, woody scents with a trace of musk.

Carry your perfume in a small fancy bottle on a chain. A little box filled with perfume cream is also nice for freshening up in the middle of the day.

If you have a decanter or atomizer with a very small neck and you want to refill it, try using a syringe. You can decant without spilling a single drop.

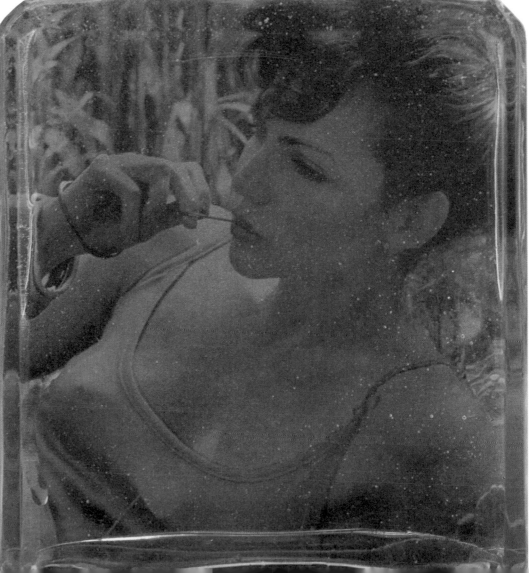

How Fragrances Are Made

Finding the right perfume is not as easy as it seems. About 2,000 types of fragrances are made. They can be divided into eight major groups:

Woody Scents have a fresh, sporty character. They are reminiscent of cedarwood, sandalwood and autumn leaves.

Mossy Scents are dominated by oakmoss.

Herbal Scents are characterized by clover and sweet grass.

Floral Scents are like gardens in bloom. You can detect violets, jasmine and lily of the valley. This group also contains some woody and fruity scents.

Spicy Scents have a sharp, slightly harsh tone underlying the flowery scent. The crusaders supposedly brought these back from Cyprus.

Leather-and-Tobacco Scents are pungent and frequently have the aroma of birch.

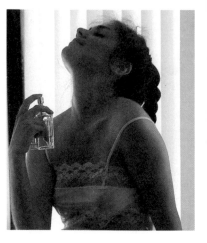

Aldehydic Scents are synthetically made, fruity aromas.

Oriental Scents smell like vanilla, myrrh and balsam.

These sultry perfumes became fashionable again several years ago.

The base material for perfume consists of extracts from blossoms and animals. These are added to synthetic products. One reason perfumes are so expensive is that manufacturers sometimes need years to develop a new scent. Another is that enormous amounts of ingredients are required to produce small amounts of fragrances. To produce approximately 2 pounds of jasmine concentrate, 5 million blossoms have to be picked, sorted and processed through a complex extraction procedure.

The animal substances in perfumes are also expensive to obtain. For example, musk comes from the sex gland of the nearly extinct musk deer.

Other animal substances in perfumes include *castoreum* and *ambergris*. Castoreum is produced by the male beaver in two tiny pouches under his stomach. It attracts female beavers. Ambergris is produced by the sperm whale as an aid to digestion.

Don't let these details spoil the pleasure you get from perfume. Animal scents by themselves may smell repugnant. When added to perfume in small quantities, they give it an exotic touch.

Perfume is a breath of luxury. Fragrance concentrate is produced from millions of blossoms. Perfume manufacturers even create enchanting scents from petroleum.

How to Wear Your Fragrance

If you dab it on sparingly, you can use perfume from early morning on. The rule that your fragrance during the day should be very light, like eau de cologne, is outdated. Woody and floral scents are especially well suited for day wear. Dab a little behind your ears. Then apply it elsewhere.

Perfume's scent unfolds best on the thin skin over the arteries. Put perfume on your wrist, in the bend of your elbow and knee, between your breasts, and on your ankles.

Your hair is also an excellent fragrance carrier. Dab perfume in the hair near your temple, or spray it directly on your hair. You can also add a few drops to the final rinse water when you wash your hair.

You can be much more extravagant when applying eau de cologne or eau de toilette. Spray yourself from head to toe. You'll find it refreshing.

Liquid perfumes evaporate quickly on very dry skin. Use a cream perfume or a perfumed body lotion instead. Or add a few drops of your favorite scent to the unperfumed body lotion that you use after bathing.

Several factors affect perfume's scent. If your perfume seems different, it may no longer be fresh. Perfume has a short shelf life after it has been opened.

Light and heat can change the scent, so be sure you store perfume in a cool, dark place.

Changes in your body can alter fragrances. Menstruation and pregnancy affect the way perfume reacts with your skin. They also affect your sense of smell, and you may find scents that you previously liked seem unpleasant. Taking medication and eating garlic, onions and very spicy foods may also change your perfume's fragrance.

The scent of the perfume unfolds as it comes in contact with your skin.

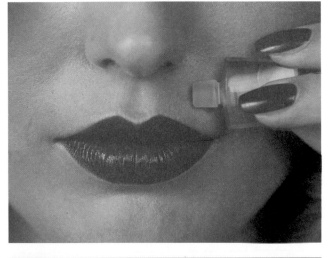

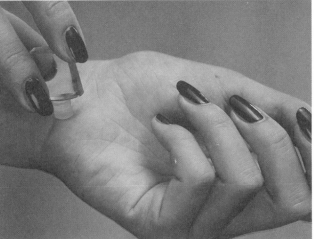

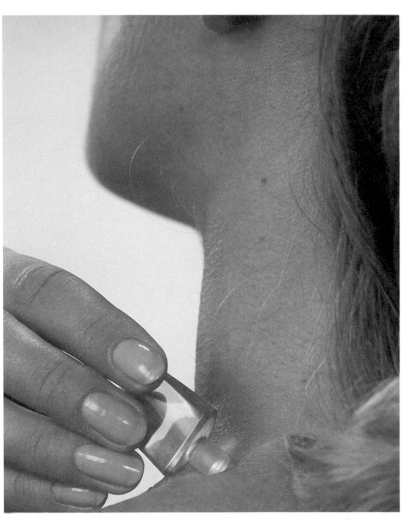

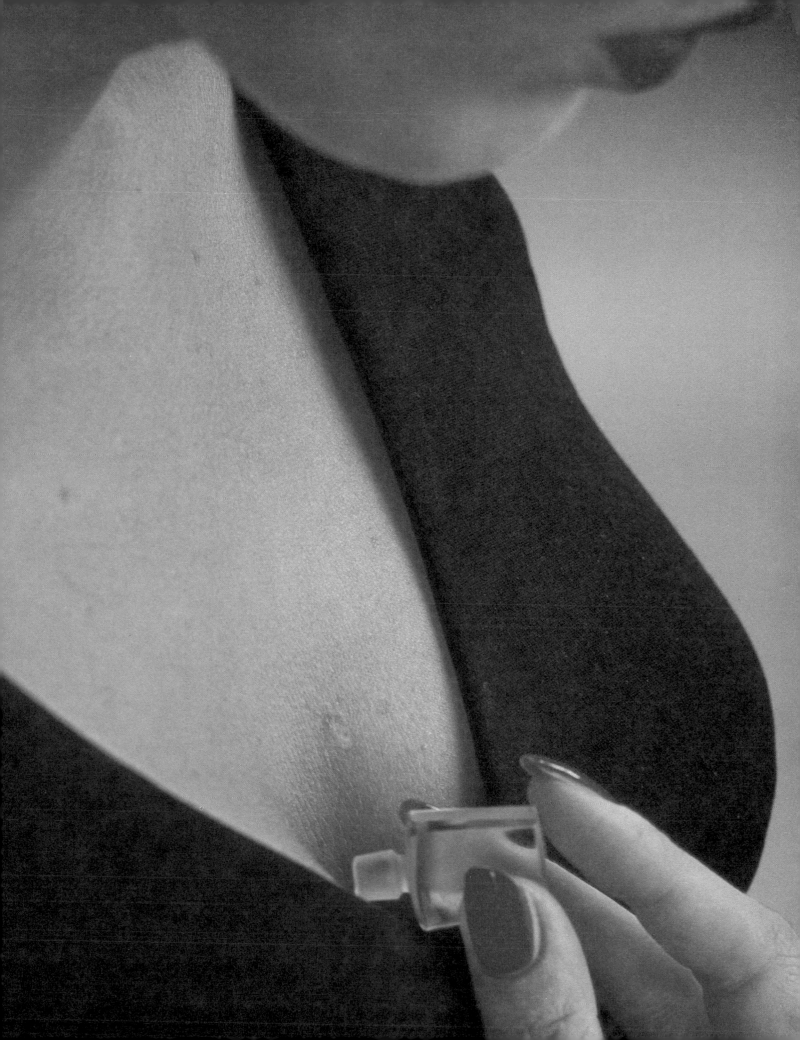

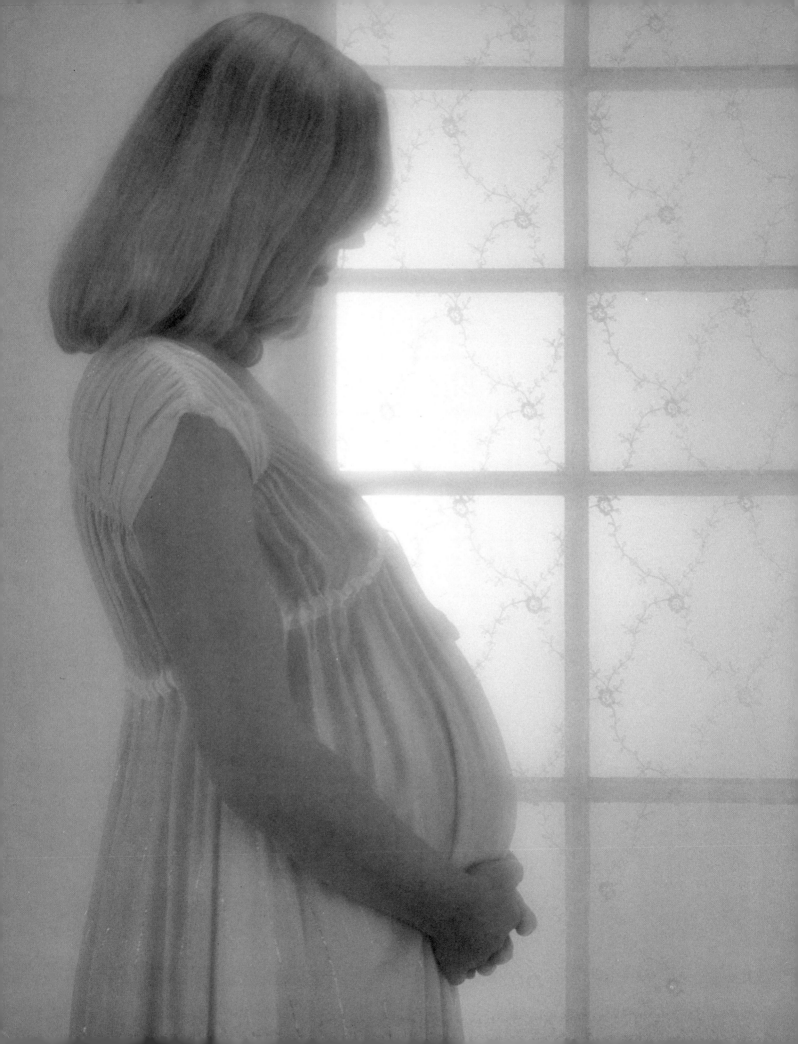

Pregnancy

You need to change your beauty program during pregnancy. Hormonal changes will significantly affect all parts of your body. Dry skin becomes drier. Acne clears up. Oily skin becomes normal. Hair tends to lose some of its luster. After giving birth, your skin and hair will return to their original condition by themselves. This may not happen with your figure. To be on the safe side, take preventive measures. Be sure to exercise and watch your diet. You'll find this will help not only your body, but also your spirits.

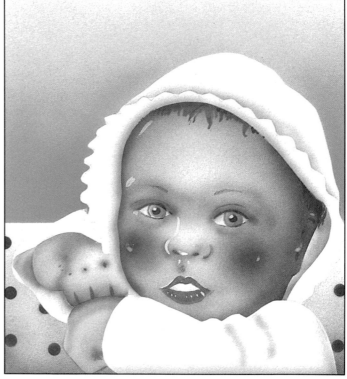

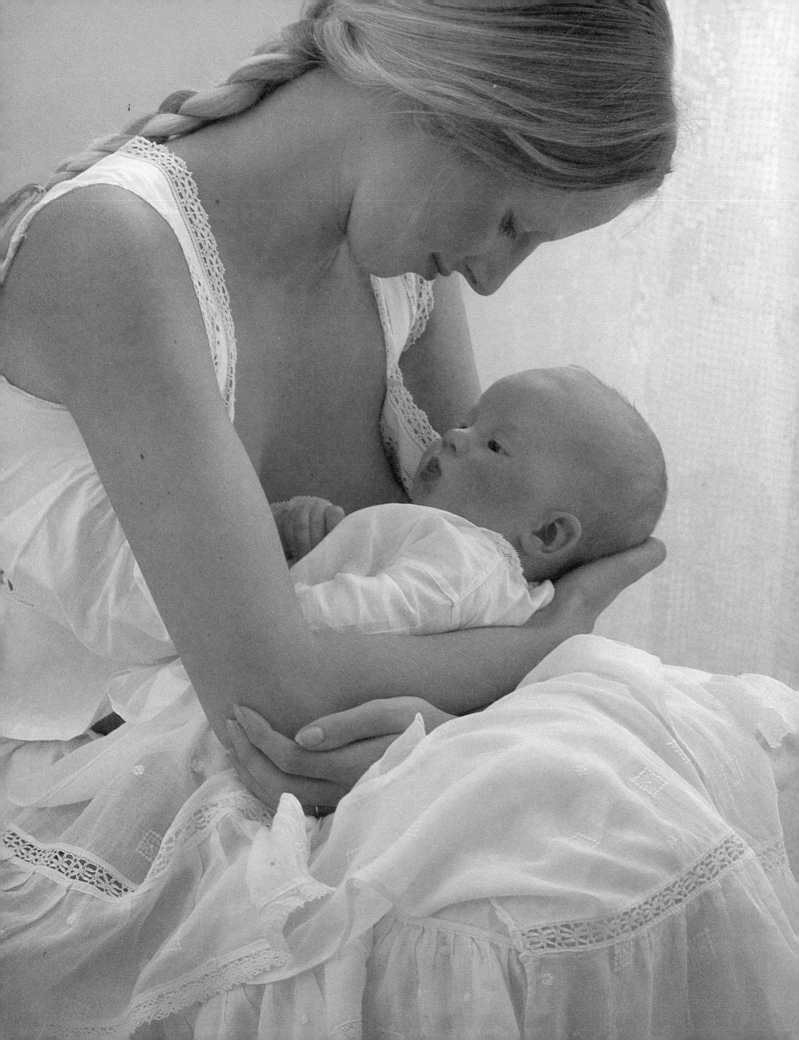

Pregnancy Can Be Beautiful

Pregnancy profoundly affects your body. Skin and hair become drier as your hormone balance changes.

The major reason for these changes is that your body produces estrogen in enormous quantities. Estrogen overwhelms other hormones, including those influencing the sebaceous glands in your skin and scalp.

Special facial care is not necessary during pregnancy. Use products formulated for your "new" skin type. Use an additional facial mask occasionally if your skin looks more tired than usual.

The one major skin problem you may have is a proliferation of brown pregnancy spots on your forehead and cheeks. You can't eliminate these spots, but you can minimize them with makeup. The discoloration is intensified by exposure to the sun. Use a sunblock when you go out during the day.

Your fingernails and toenails may become brittle during these months. A daily massage with oil may help.

Your hair will also become drier. Simply switch to products appropriate for your hair's condition at this time.

Your stomach and bosom need special care. The natural elasticity of muscles and ligaments usually ensures that women regain their slender figures after delivery. Nevertheless, additional measures can help.

Oil your stomach morning and evening. This will help keep skin supple. However, there is no evidence that any type of oil or cream will help prevent stretch marks. These are an inevitable side effect of pregnancy.

The bosom becomes heavier during the second month of pregnancy. Even if you do not usually wear a bra, use one during pregnancy. It will provide additional support.

Be sure to exercise every day. This will tone your muscles and lift your spirits. Don't be overly concerned by what happens to your body during these months. Your hormone balance will readjust after delivery and your skin and hair will return to the condition they were in before you became pregnant. Your figure should do the same.

Good nutrition is a must during this time. You should eat a well-balanced diet that includes plenty of fresh fruit and vegetables, milk products, meat and poultry, and grains. Whole-grain bread is also highly recommended. It supplies important vitamins and stimulates digestion.

Your caloric intake during pregnancy should be adjusted according to the recommendations of your physician.

You may have trouble sleeping, especially during the last three months. Try changing positions frequently.

If you find yourself feeling abnormally tired, you may be anemic. Anemia occurs when the body produces more blood serum than corpuscles. This frequently happens during pregnancy. It can be rectified with iron supplements. Your doctor can give you a prescription.

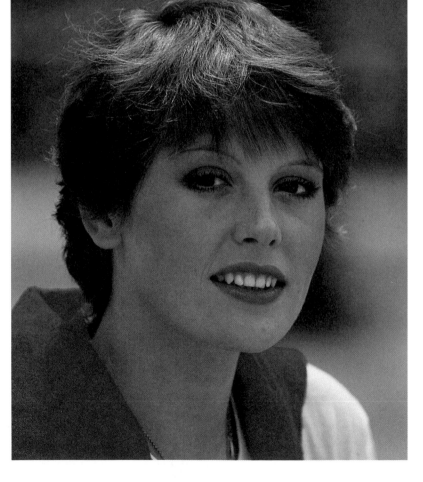

Pregnancy changes the hormone balance of your body, which affects skin and hair. You must change your beauty program during this time.

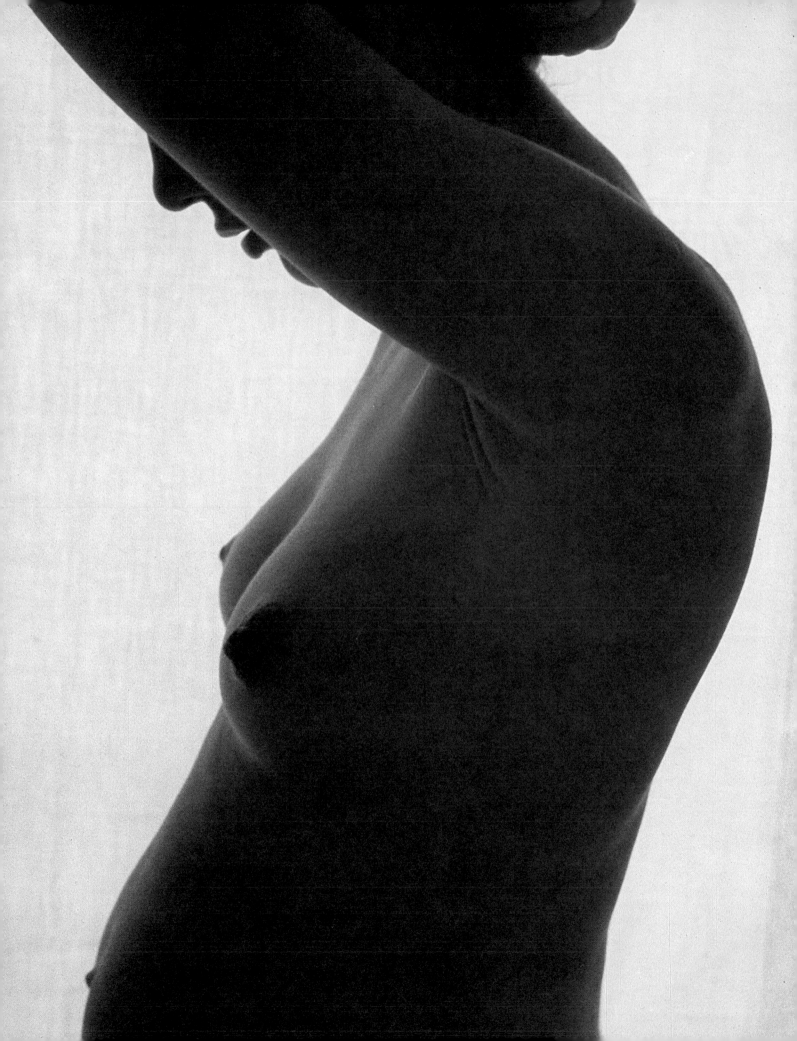

Fitness During Pregnancy

Being pregnant doesn't mean you have to change your entire lifestyle. You should feel fit and fine every day if you follow a few rules.

If you work, find a quiet corner and elevate your legs for a few minutes at the end of the day. Relax and take a deep breath. A refreshing cup of tea helps, too.

You can also unwind by using cold compresses or by putting your arms and elbows in cold water. A lukewarm bath is also refreshing. It is especially beneficial for your legs and feet, which tend to swell during pregnancy.

You can also make your legs feel better by massaging them and elevating them whenever possible.

If you have problems with backaches, try these exercises. Kneel on the floor, arch your back like a cat, then straighten it again. Or lie on your back, push the small of your back toward the floor, then relax. Repeat these exercises 5 times, working up to 25.

Get as much fresh air as possible while you're pregnant. Walking is good exercise and will give you additional energy. Don't forget to use a sunblock.

Swimming is an excellent activity during pregnancy. It relieves muscle aches and strengthens the muscular system, which helps minimize problems during delivery.

Bicycling is permitted, too, but avoid long trips.

The more varied your menus are, the greater the possibility your body is getting what it needs.

Be sure to eat enough bulk and fiber. These help regulate the digestive system. They are found in grains, fruits and vegetables. You can also add fibrous foods to other dishes. For example, bran is delicious on cereal and salads.

If you are overweight, starving off a few pounds won't solve anything. To keep weight off permanently, you have to change your eating habits.

You can do this gradually. Try eating dessert only when you really crave something sweet. Substitute fruit for candy or ice cream when you want to get a quick lift during the day.

Don't force yourself to eat foods you don't like just because you think they're good for you. Build your new eating habits around healthful foods you enjoy. Otherwise, you will feel so deprived that you will either abandon your new food plan or binge on the replacement foods.

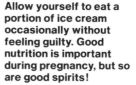

Allow yourself to eat a portion of ice cream occasionally without feeling guilty. Good nutrition is important during pregnancy, but so are good spirits!

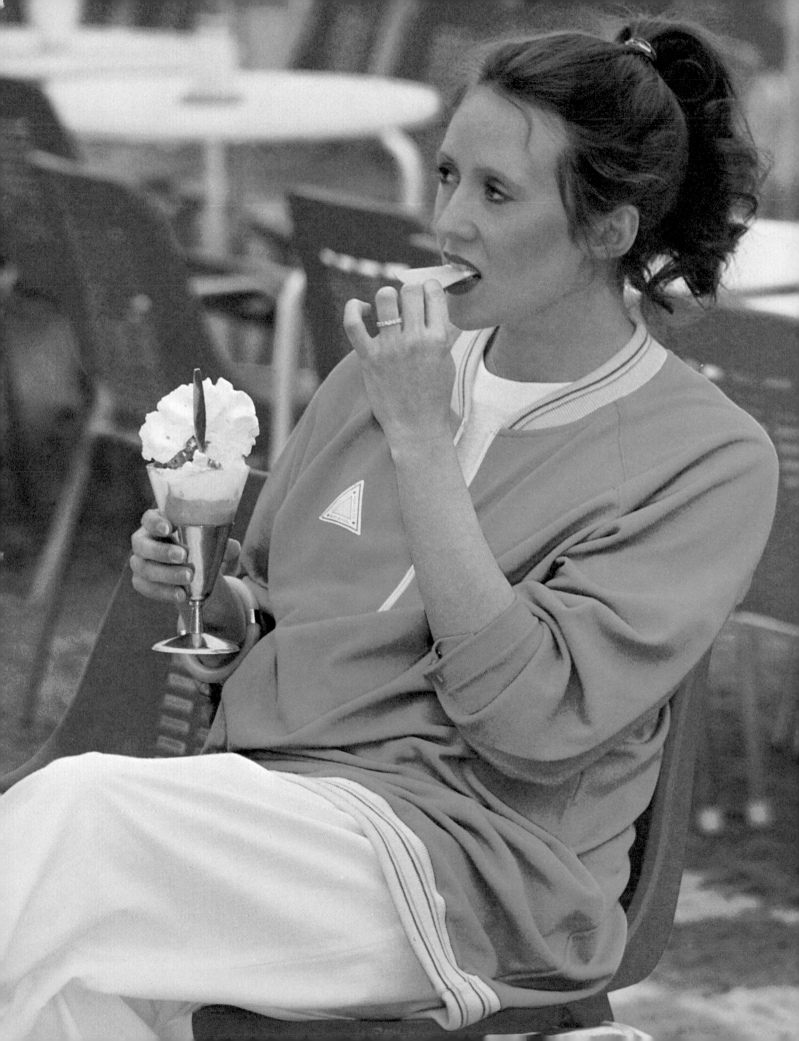

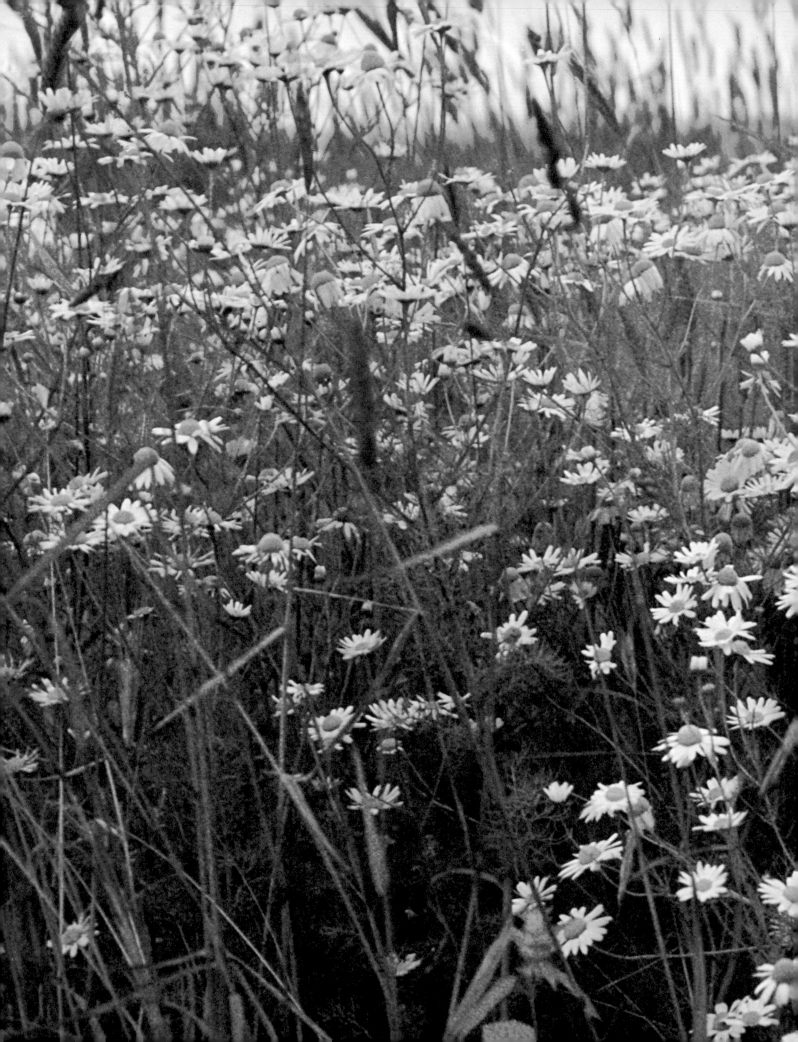

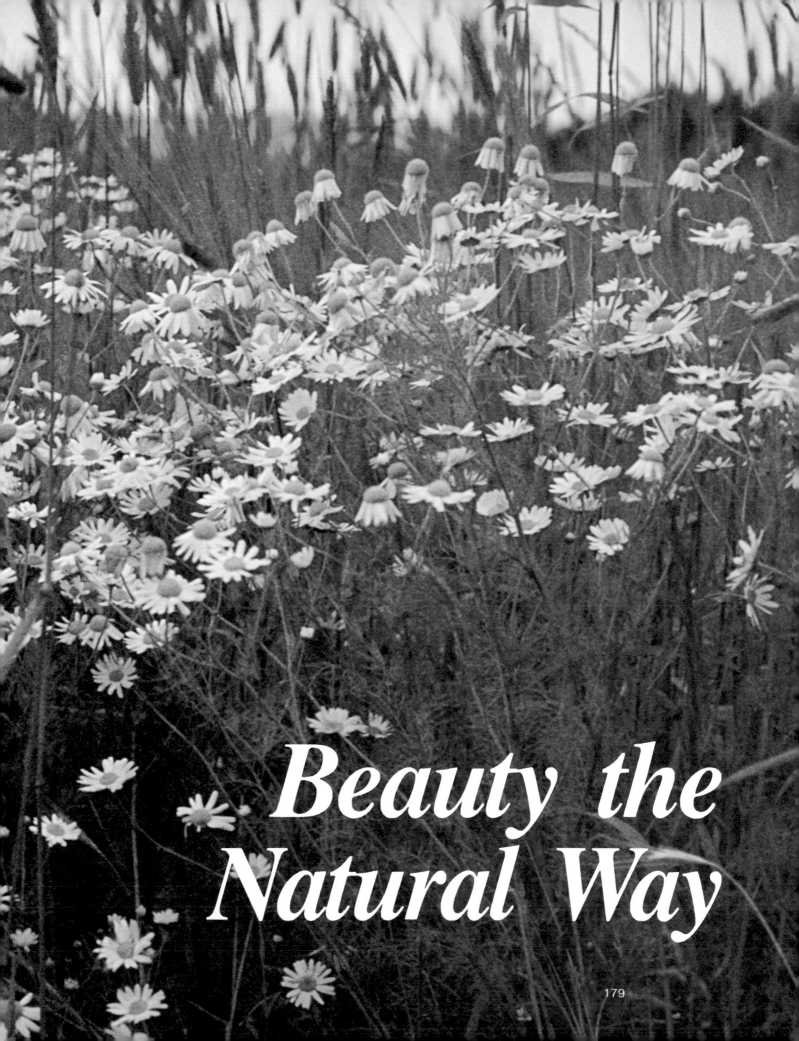

Beauty the Natural Way

G

reen meadows, waving cornfields, abundant gardens. They evoke a vision of a more healthful life. You can have this kind of life. It's easier than you think. All you have to do is change a few habits. Don't use so many packaged and processed foods. Eat fresh foods instead. Don't look for a pill to relieve every minor ache and pain. Try a few simple home remedies first. Don't rely totally on expensive cosmetic products. See what preparations you can make yourself from natural ingredients.

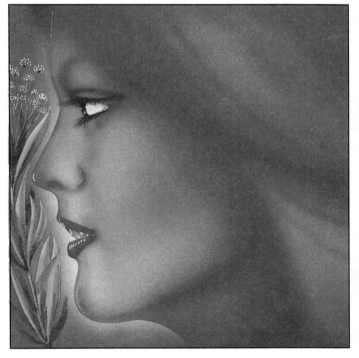

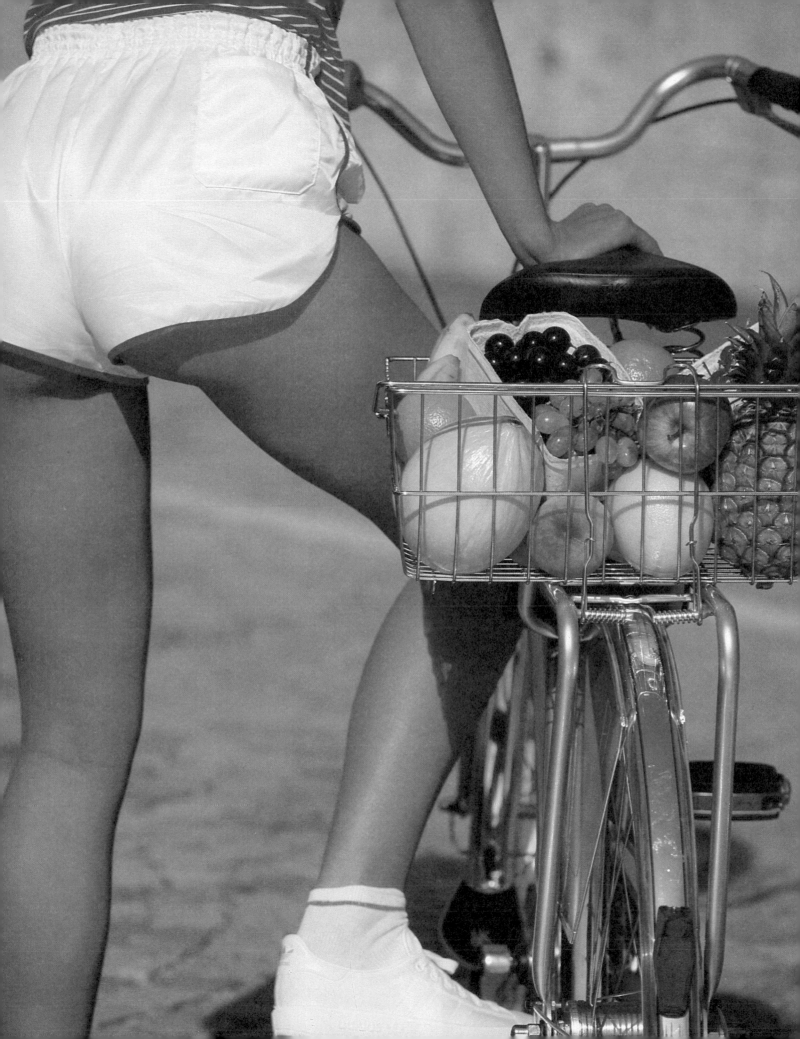

Eating the Natural Way

Proper nutrition is important for beauty. Your daily meals should supply your body with all the protein, vitamins, trace elements and minerals it needs. You can help ensure this by following these guidelines:

Buy Fresh Foods—Canned foods should be used only rarely if you want to follow a truly *natural* regimen. Fresh ingredients are much more healthful.

Store Foods Properly—Fresh foods should be refrigerated. If you need to store them for long periods of time, freeze them. Foods lose some vitamins and minerals if they are not stored properly.

Never Soak Fruit and Vegetables—The longer these foods are in water, the more nutrients they lose. Just rinse them off thoroughly.

Don't Mince Vegetables—It may be fashionable to cut vegetables into tiny pieces, but mincing vegetables increases the surface area through which vital nutrients can be lost during cooking. Leave vegetables you plan to cook in one piece or cut them into several large pieces. You can mince them at the table.

Potatoes should not be peeled before cooking. Their skins are nutritious, and reduce the loss of vitamins and minerals during cooking.

Cook with a Timer—The shorter the cooking time, the better. Make sure every cooked vegetable is somewhat crunchy. This ensures that important nutrients are intact.

Cook with as little water as possible. Cover only half the contents of a pot or pan and use lids that close tightly. Let steam cook the food.

Serve Hot Foods Immediately—Well-organized cooks make sure every dish is ready at the same time. This ensures that meals provide maximum nutrition. Foods lose vitamins and minerals if they sit too long at room temperature.

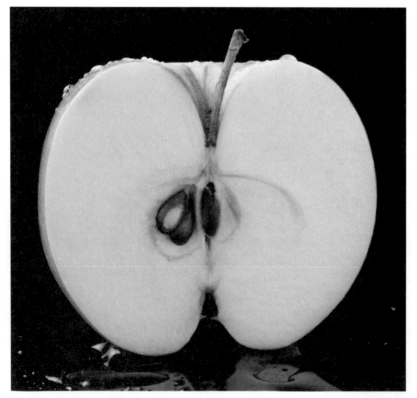

Apples are beautifiers. They are rich in vitamins and fiber.

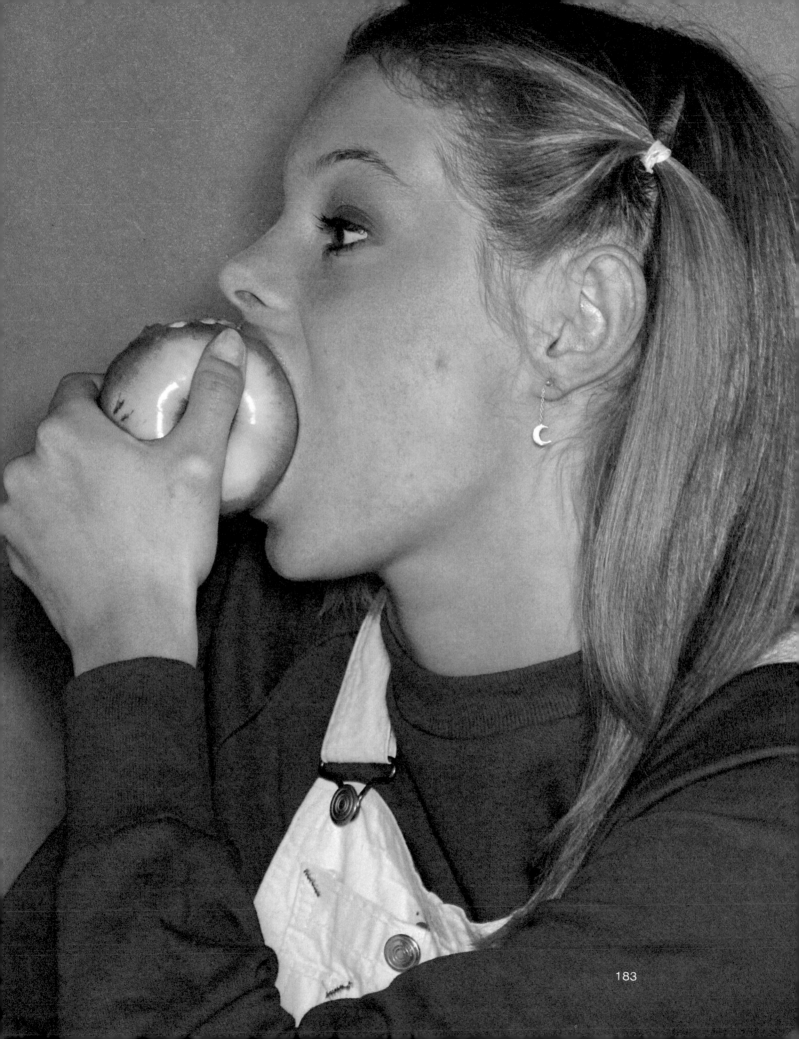

Natural Cosmetics—Grains

Try a new 1-week beauty program. Whole-wheat flour, wheat germ and wheat germ oils are excellent beauty aids.

The grain beauty plan starts with washing your face every morning with a paste made from whole-wheat flour. Every other evening, take a wheat-paste bath and apply a grain mask to your face.

If you have rough, leathery skin, use a facial scrub before starting this treatment.

The program will be more effective if you also take frequent walks and visit a sauna twice during the week.

Wheat-Paste Beauty Bath—

This is especially recommended if you have oily or blemished skin.

You'll need a small muslin bag that can be tied at the top and hung under a faucet. A muslin diaper or a handkerchief will work, too. Take the corners and tie them together with a string. The more porous the material, the more wheat-flour paste can pass through to pamper your skin.

If you have oily or blemished skin, put 2 tablespoons each whole-wheat flour, chamomile blossoms and lemon balm into the bag. Tie it, hang it under the bathtub faucet and turn on the water. When the tub is full, get in and remove the bag. Squeeze it until the milky paste penetrates the material. Gently massage blemished skin with it. Soak in the wheat-paste water 20 minutes. Then wrap yourself in a bath towel and go to bed without drying off.

If you have dry skin, put 2 tablespoons whole-wheat flour and 2 tablespoons powdered milk in a bag and let water run over it. When you get in the tub, massage your skin with the bag. Dry yourself afterward and apply body lotion.

Grain Masks—The best time to apply this type of mask is when you take a bath. Don't cover your eyes and lips. If your neck has blemishes, always treat it along with your face.

For normal to oily skin, mix 1 tablespoon whole-wheat flour with 2 tablespoons buttermilk. Or mix 1 tablespoon wheat germ with 1 tablespoon water and 1/2 teaspoon fruit vinegar.

Apply the paste to your face and allow it to congeal. After bathing, rub yourself gently with a clean, damp washcloth. Rinse off with water and apply night cream.

Wheat-germ oil is an effective cosmetic oil. It keeps skin from becoming leathery.

For dry skin, mix 1 tablespoon wheat germ with 1 tablespoon wheat germ oil. Or mix 2 tablespoons oatmeal with 2 tablespoons buttermilk. You can also use 2 tablespoons oatmeal with 2 tablespoons chamomile tea or thinned chamomile extract.

Let the mask dry. After bathing, press a clean, wet washcloth on the dried mask. Soak the mask without rubbing too much. Then wipe your face gently and rinse with lukewarm water. Apply night cream.

Wheat-Paste Facial Wash—

Put whole-wheat flour in a saucer and add a little water. Stir until it becomes thick and sticky. Gently massage your face with the mixture. This removes dead skin cells, makes skin smoother and stimulates circulation. Afterward, rinse off the paste under running, lukewarm-to-cool water. Apply moisturizing cream.

Because paste made from whole-wheat flour removes natural oils, this facial wash formula should be used only for normal, oily or blemished skin. If you have dry skin, use a paste made from powdered milk.

You can buy whole-wheat flour, wheat germ and oatmeal in health food stores. Lemon balm is available in stores specializing in herbs. You can find skin treatments with wheat-germ oil in health food stores.

For the baths and washes you'll need approximately 9 ounces whole-wheat flour, 3-1/2 ounces chamomile blossoms and 3-1/2 ounces lemon balm. If you have dry skin, you'll need 9 ounces whole-wheat flour and approximately 9 ounces powdered milk.

For the mask, buy approximately 3-1/2 ounces whole-wheat flour. If you have dry skin, buy 3-1/2 ounces oatmeal or wheat germ.

Apply grain masks while bathing. Steam makes them more effective.

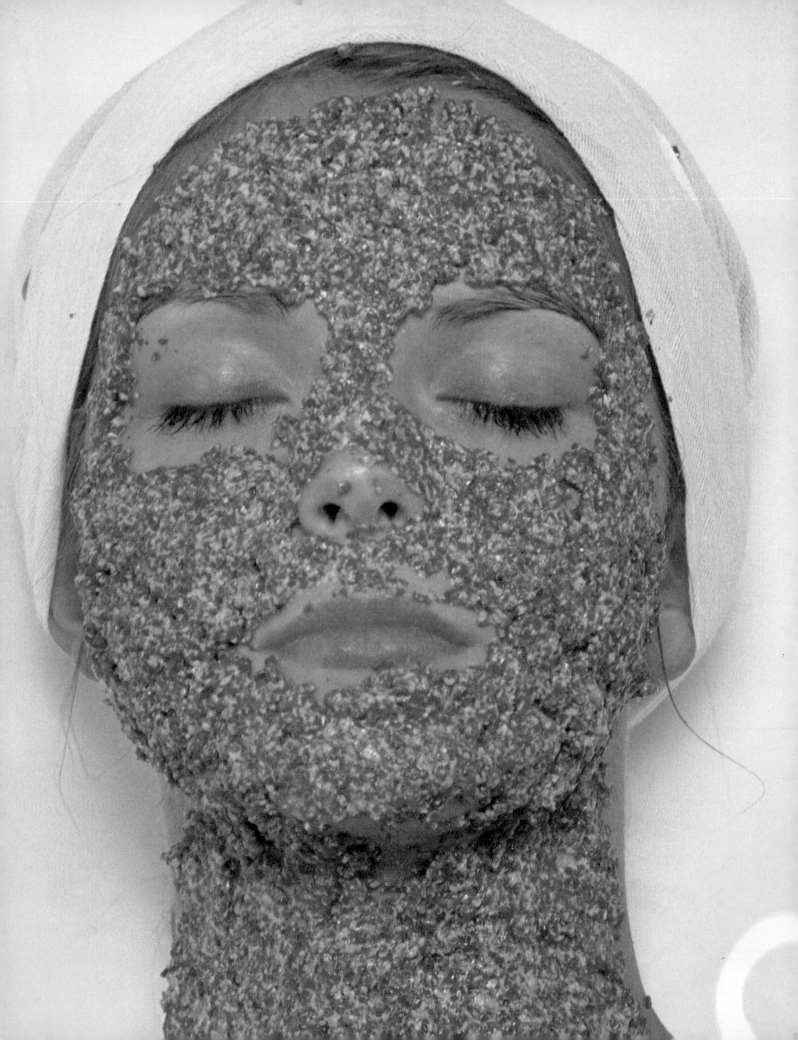

Natural Cosmetics—Herbs

If you are tired, nervous, have muscle pains or difficulties sleeping, you undoubtedly have beauty problems. Why not try some herbal remedies? Herbal teas, compresses and herbal baths can make you look and feel better.

Herbs affect not only your skin, but your entire body when you bathe. The vapors are especially soothing to your nose, throat and lungs.

Herbal baths should be hot, but not uncomfortably so. You should take these baths only twice a week. People with high blood pressure or circulatory problems should not take herbal baths at all.

Arnica eases pain and constriction in tired legs. It is also helpful in healing slight abrasions. You can buy arnica tincture in health food stores. To make a compress, pour 1 cup boiling water over 1 teaspoon arnica tincture. Let it steep 10 minutes. Or mix 1 tablespoon arnica tincture with 1 cup warm water.

Soak muslin, cotton or linen cloth in the arnica solution. Wrap the cloth around your legs. Put hand towels over the cloth. Use tape or safety pins to keep them in place. Lie down with your legs elevated for 30 minutes.

Be sure to keep arnica tincture away from children. It

Pour 2 cups boiling water over a handful of blossoms. Hold your face over the steam. Drape a towel over your head to hold the moisture and vapors. When the preparation cools, add another 2 cups boiling water. Again put your face over the steam until the brew cools.

Herbs can help relax and beautify you.

Chamomile and Oak Bark inhibit the development of red, splotchy veins. To make a compress, add 1 teaspoon oak bark to 1 pint hot water (2

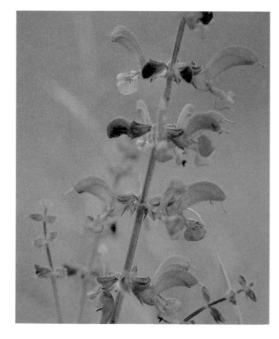

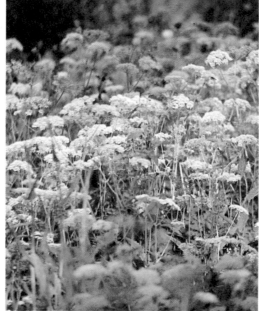

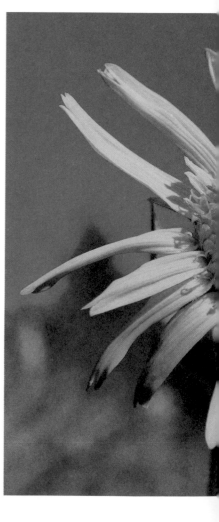

Soak in the tub 5 to 10 minutes. Relax afterward in a warm bed.

Individual herbs can be used to treat specific problems.

can be harmful if ingested.
Chamomile is beneficial for sensitive, blemished skin. It works most effectively when you use it to steam your face.

Five herbs for beauty include, from left, sage, yarrow, arnica, rosemary and shave grass. Even dried herbs should be used within one year after harvesting.

cups). Simmer 10 to 15 minutes. Add 1 teaspoon chamomile. Turn off heat. Let solution simmer 10 to 15 minutes. Soak cotton cloth in the solution. Put cloth over veins. Leave it in place 5 minutes. Repeat every day for at least 6 months.

Rosemary leaves can soothe skin. You can use rosemary as a tea or in your bath. To make tea, add 1 heaping teaspoon rosemary to 1 cup cold water. Bring to a boil. Strain immediately.

For an herbal bath, add 2 ounces (by weight) of rosemary to 1 quart water (4 cups). Bring to a boil. Turn off heat and let rosemary steep 30 minutes.

Strain and pour into bath water.

Rosemary is refreshing and energizing. Don't use it in your bath before going to bed. You'll be wide awake.

Store dried herbs in tightly closed containers in a cool, dark place.

Sage calms the nervous system. It works well as a strong tea. Pour 1 cup boiling water over 1 teaspoon sage leaves. Let it steep 15 minutes. If you have a sensitive stomach, eat something before drinking the tea.

put 2 teaspoons dried shave grass in 1 cup cold water. Let it steep 12 hours. Or you can bring it to a boil. Turn off heat and let shave grass steep 10 minutes, then strain it. If you make a compress, soak muslin or cotton cloth in the cooled brew. Put cloth over veins. Leave it in place at least 5 minutes. Repeat several times a week for at least 6 months.

Yarrow inhibits infections and is especially good for oily and blemished skin. Try it in your bath. Put 2 handfuls of yarrow tea in 1 quart of water (4 cups). Bring to a boil. Turn off heat and let yarrow steep 15 minutes. Strain it into bath water.

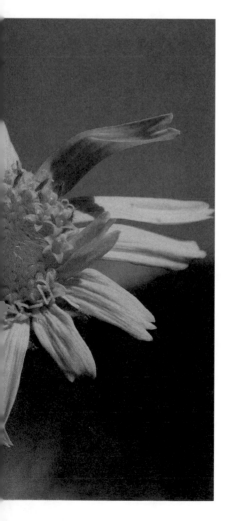
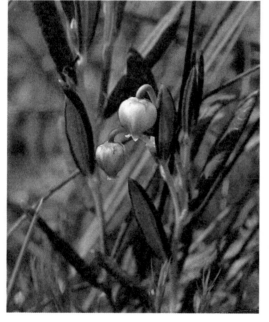
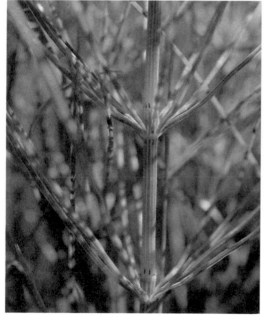

Shave Grass alleviates splotchy veins. It contains an acid that supposedly improves the elasticity of connective tissue. Shave grass is effective as a tea or compress. For either,

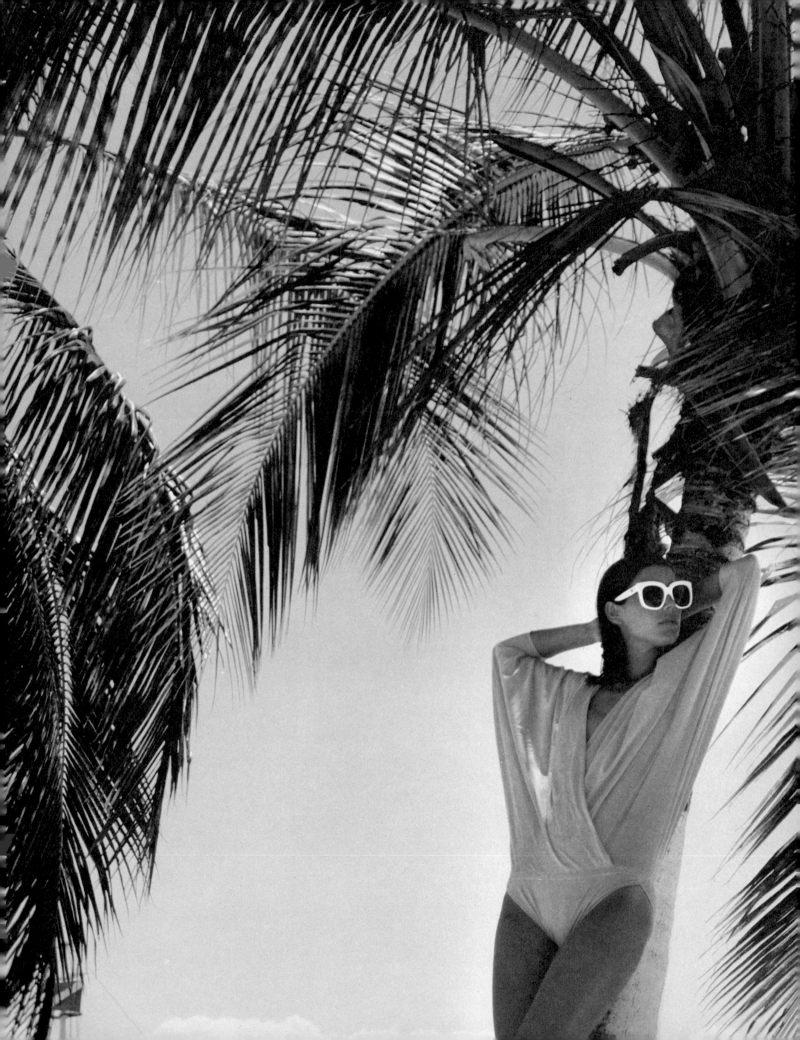

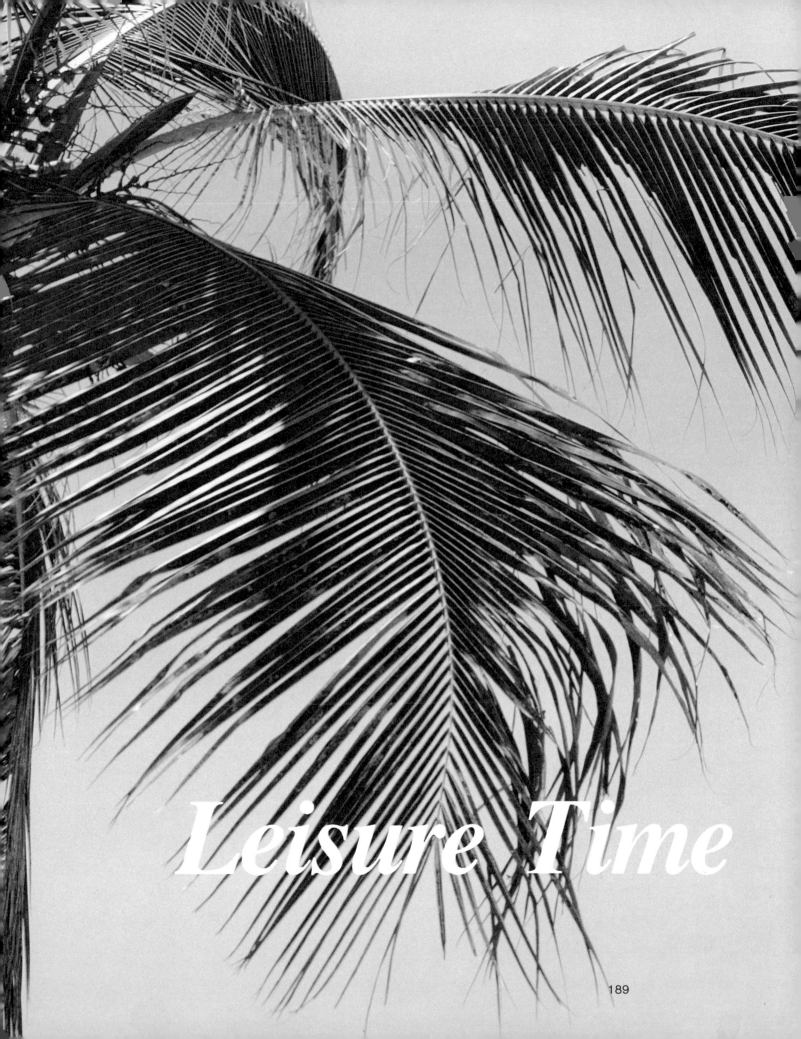

Leisure Time

*U*p to this point, you have learned what you can do to be well-groomed from head to toe. You've seen many techniques and products that can make you more attractive. This final chapter is devoted to your leisure time. This kind of time—time for yourself—is a beauty aid that even the best cosmetic products can't compete with. These products work only on the outside. Leisure time works on your inner self. You can use it to create serenity and a sense 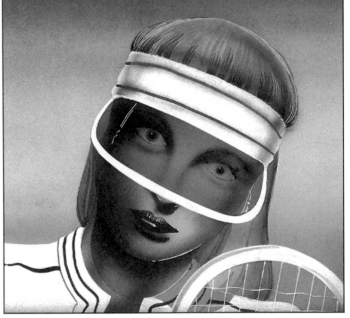 of well-being. This peace of mind makes you beautiful inside and out. So be sure to take part of every day as leisure time for yourself—time away from family, daily pressures and stress. Pamper yourself with an extravagant breakfast or a long telephone conversation with a dear friend. Or just daydream quietly for 5 minutes. These things help make you pretty, too. Make them a permanent part of your beauty program.

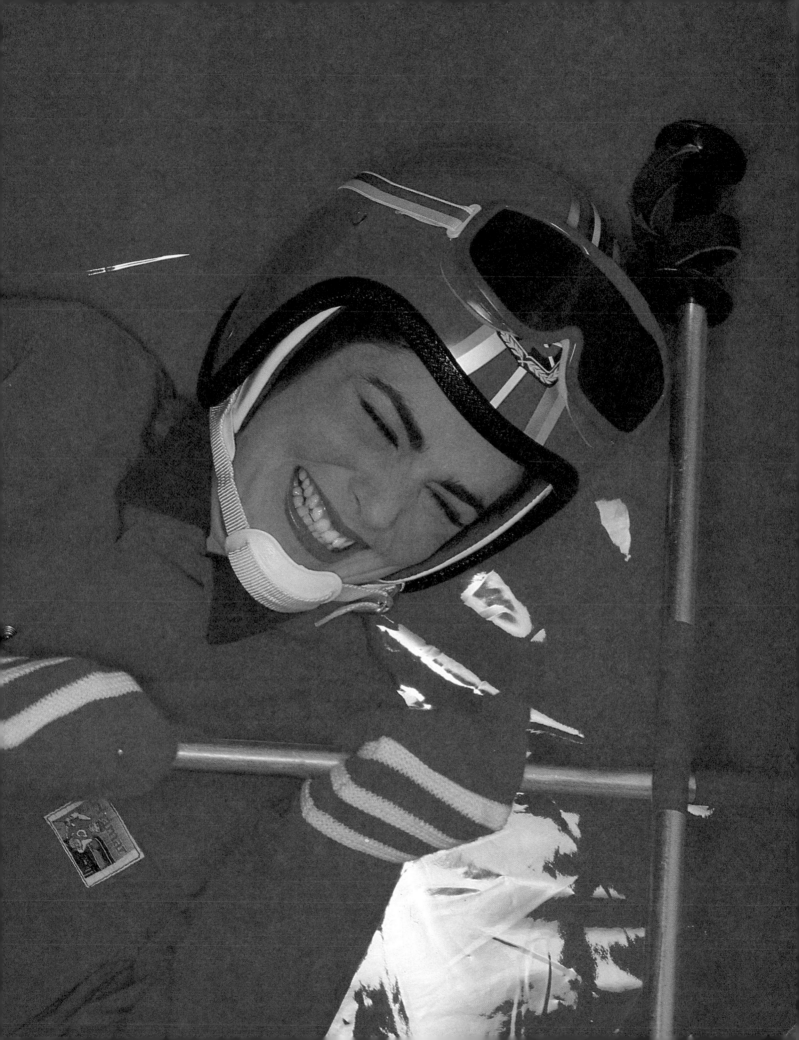

You and the Sun

Many people feel a suntan is beautiful. The problem with this attitude is that it ignores the fact that the sun damages skin. Long-term exposure, even without burning, causes skin to age prematurely, resulting in loss of elasticity, wrinkling and drying. Exposure from childhood to adulthood can lead to precancerous conditions and skin cancer.

The body has two defenses against the sun. The first is increased pigmentation. When skin has been exposed to the sun for a long time, cells produce additional *melanin,* a dark pigment that offers some protection against the sun's ultraviolet rays. This pigment is what makes us look tan. The second defense mechanism is a strengthening of the outer layer of skin. Increased cell activity helps form a natural filter to protect skin against ultraviolet light.

However, these defenses are not sufficient. The skin needs additional help. Numerous products are available that provide extra protection against the effects of the sun. These products are called *sunscreens* and *sunblocks.* Applied properly, they filter some or all of the sun's harmful ultraviolet rays.

It is important to remember that suntan lotion will not protect your skin against the sun's harmful effects. They contain mostly emollients and oils. These keep your skin moist, but do not block any ultraviolet rays.

Sunscreens and Sunblocks—Sunscreens filter some of the sun's ultraviolet rays. Each sunscreen has a *sun protection factor,* a number from 2 to 15 that is printed on the bottle. The number indicates how much additional protection the product provides. Sun protection factor 3, for example, means you have three times your natural skin protection against the sun. A product with a sun protection factor of 15 will afford almost complete protection against the effects of ultraviolet rays.

Sunblocks filter nearly all of

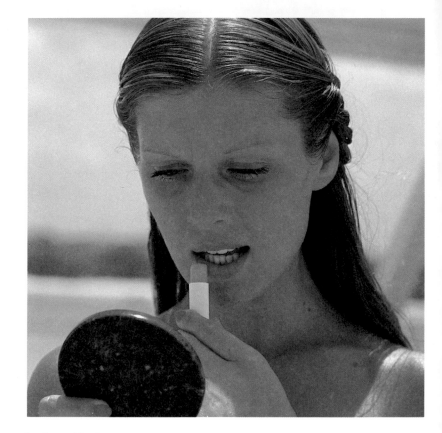

Apply sunblock or sunscreen frequently to your lips, eyes and nose. They are very easily sunburned.

the sun's rays. They are opaque, and include ingredients such as zinc oxide paste.

Which sunscreen or sunblock you choose will depend upon several factors. If you are going swimming or water skiing, use a water-resistant or waterproof product. The most beneficial sunscreens and sunblocks are those containing a chemical called *para-aminobenzoic acid,* or *PABA*. If you have dry skin, use a moisture-based sunscreen or sunblock with PABA. If you have oily skin, use an alcohol-based product with PABA.

If you are one of the small number of people who is allergic to PABA, get a cinnamate-based or benzophenone-based sunscreen or sunblock.

The most healthful thing to do regarding the sun is to avoid exposure as much as possible. Use a sunblock when you will be outside any length of time. Wear pretty hats and silky, long-sleeved blouses.

Artificial Tanning Products—These include tanning creams and tablets. These preparations are usually not satisfactory. They produce uneven coloration, and can turn the skin an unpleasant orange or bronze color. If tanning creams are applied by hand, they can stain your palms.

Tanning booths and salons have become popular the last several years. You should avoid them, however. They can severely damage your skin and can cause eye burns.

Protecting Yourself from the Sun

If you insist on sunbathing, follow these guidelines:

1. Be sure to wear a sunblock or a sunscreen with a very high sun protection factor. If you burn at all, you should use a sunblock and allow yourself to tan very slowly. Remember that if you sunbathe near water, you will also be exposed to sun reflecting off the water, which multiplies the harmful effects. Wind and high altitudes also intensify the effects of the sun. Don't forget that you can get sunburned on cloudy days.

2. Be especially careful to protect your face. Make sure your lips are covered with lip balm containing PABA.

3. If you tend to get freckles, use a sunblock.

4. Don't use perfume or eau de cologne. You'll develop pigment spots.

5. The skin around your eyes is very thin. Apply a sunscreen or sunblock liberally to this area. You should also wear sunglasses with large lenses.

6. When you lie in the sun, put cotton pads with cream on your eyelids.

7. Be sure to use a sunscreen or sunblock on and behind your ears. They are very sensitive to the sun.

8. Your nose burns more quickly than the rest of your face because the sun strikes it at a steeper angle. Reapply sunscreen or sunblock every 20 minutes.

9. If you enjoy water sports, use water-resistant skin preparations. These preparations protect for as long as 40 minutes of continuous water exposure. Waterproof products are also available. They protect for as long as 80 minutes of continuous water exposure. Always shower afterward and apply body lotion or moisturizing cream.

10. Never lie dripping wet in the sun. It makes your skin too susceptible to damage.

Be sure to use a sunblock or a sunscreen with a very high sun protection factor.

11. Hair is as sun-sensitive as skin. Too much exposure bleaches your hair and makes it dull and brittle. Wear a cap when swimming and a hat or scarf when sunbathing. Hair cream also offers some protection against the sun. When you wash your hair, use a creme rinse or conditioner. Be sure to dry your wet hair in the shade.

12. When you sit in the sun, drink plenty of fluids. If you're hungry, eat only light meals. Try fruit, vegetables, yogurt, cheese or fish.

After sunbathing, use creams and lotions formulated for sunburned skin. These preparations also replace moisture and minimize peeling. They can't undo damage resulting from severe sunburn, however. Your skin will peel no matter what you use.

If you realize you've been in the sun too long, go inside immediately. Moving into the shade is not enough. You're still exposed to ultraviolet rays.

If blisters appear, see a doctor. Don't expose the burned places to the sun until the last trace of redness is gone.

Skin Care in Winter

Winter is an enemy of beauty. Outside, cold and wind attack your skin. Inside, dry heat robs your skin of moisture, making it feel uncomfortably tight. To keep your skin from looking tired and drawn, you have to give it special treatment.

Every type of skin needs additional moisture during the winter. Apply cream several times a day, especially if your skin feels tight.

Remember that you can get a sunburn even in winter. Be especially careful if you're going to take a skiing vacation and spend a lot of time in the snow.

If outside temperatures are very low, use a cream formulated to protect your skin against the cold in addition to your day cream. These special creams insulate skin beautifully because they don't contain water.

Makeup is especially recommended during the winter because it helps protect skin. Start by applying cream with extra moisturizers. Then put on foundation and cover with powder. This will help keep skin warm and prevent it from losing too much moisture.

The eye area is the most sensitive part of the face. Skin dries out quickly and is susceptible to wrinkles. Be sure to put cream around your eyes and on your eyelids every day.

You will also have to pay special attention to your lips in cold weather. They can quickly become chapped and rough. Use lip balm with PABA and lipsticks with moisturizers.

In the evening, skin should be cleansed as gently as possible. Use mild cleansers and a toner containing little or no alcohol. Then apply moisturizing cream that has additional oils.

One problem you may have in winter is the proliferation of small red veins on your face. These occur because veins contract when you go outside in the cold, then expand when you return inside, where it's warm. Sometimes small veins are not strong enough to take this constant contraction and expansion. They break, forming a red splotch under the skin. Using moisturizers and makeup can help protect your skin to some extent. Scarves that you can wrap around the lower part of your face will also insulate skin from temperature changes.

If you participate in winter sports, apply makeup beforehand. It will help protect your skin from the cold, wind and sun.

You'll encounter other problems if you take a vacation that involves winter sports. The combination of sun, snow and wind can ruin the strongest skin. Always use a sunblock and a lip balm with PABA when you go outside. Do this even on cloudy days. No matter how stormy it looks, you're still exposed to the sun's ultraviolet rays.

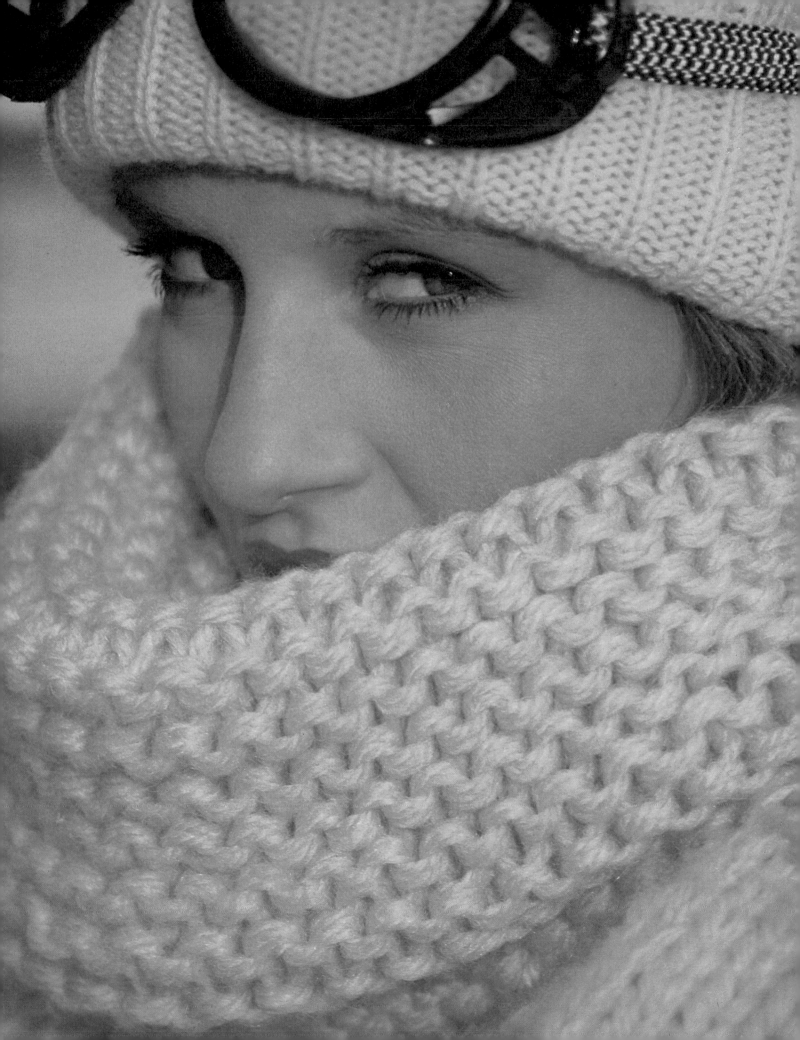

Sauna

Saunas can be healthful and beautifying. As you perspire, the outer skin layer expands and dead skin is loosened. Skin becomes smoother and looks tighter. Circulation increases, making skin rosier and more elastic.

However, people with cardiovascular problems should check with their physicians before taking saunas.

Several techniques can make your sauna even more effective:

Take a warm shower before your first trip into the sauna. Then rub your body with a massage cream or do a dry massage with a brush. This enhances the deep-cleansing effect of the sauna.

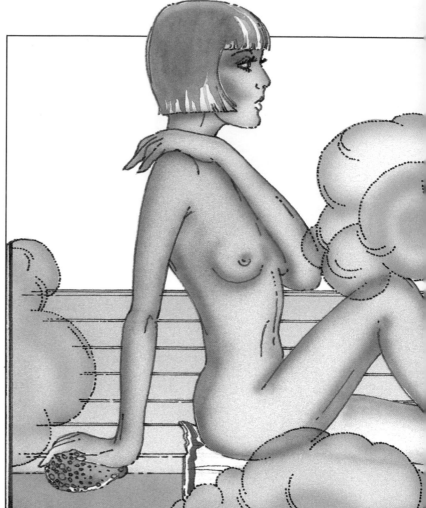

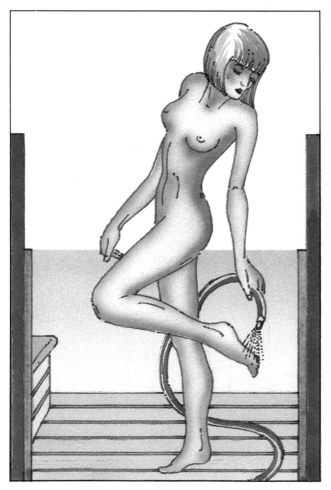

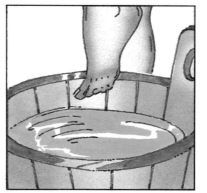

You increase the effects of the sauna by following a few guidelines.

Cleanse your face thoroughly. Use a facial scrub if you have oily or blemished skin.

Apply a conditioner to your hair before entering the sauna. The heat will make it penetrate your hair deeply. Don't wear a cap or wrap your head tightly in a towel. Much of your body heat escapes through the top of your head. If you prevent heat from escaping, it builds up in your body and can make you ill.

Saunas can be healthful and relaxing. They will relieve minor muscle aches after exercise.

Dry yourself thoroughly before going into the sauna. This will make you perspire more quickly. A warm footbath

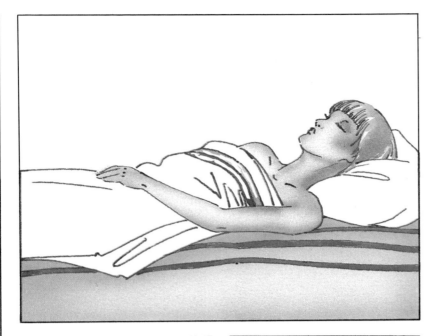

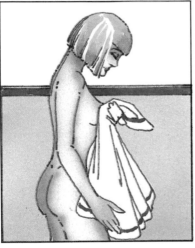

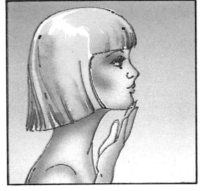

before your first trip to the sauna and after each cooling-off period helps, too.

In the sauna, lie on the middle or upper bench, where it is warmer. Move to the lowest bench when you get too hot. Be sure you lie down or sit with your legs stretched out on the bench the entire time you're in the sauna. Dangling your legs over the side makes your heart and circulatory system work too hard.

The first 3 or 4 times you take a sauna, stay in only 8 to 10 minutes before cooling off. Get up slowly or you may become dizzy.

Let your body cool off gradually. Then get in the shower and gently spray yourself. Start with your feet or arms and move toward your heart. If you start to feel cold, begin the second cycle. Return to the sauna for another 8 to 10 minutes. Then cool off again. You can repeat this procedure 3 or 4 times.

Alcohol is prohibited during and after a sauna. It forces your kidneys and circulatory system to work too hard and can be dangerous.

Saunas should always be taken after you've finished heavy activity for the day. It will relax you and ease muscle aches. Even swimming is not recommended after a sauna.

Sports

The nicest way to stay pretty and healthy is through sports. You look prettier because sports tone your muscles, condition your cardiovascular system and increase circulation to your skin. They are also an ideal way to combat stress.

First, find the sport you like best. Second, check out your exercise program with your doctor before you begin. Third, be sure you warm up before doing any exercise that increases your heart rate. You should spend at least 5 minutes doing stretches and slow-paced exercises before doing any aerobic exercise. You should also spend at least 5 minutes cooling down after strenuous exercise. Gradually reduce the intensity of your movements to help muscles relax.

You should eat lightly when exercising. Try fruit, yogurt and cheese.

Swimming is the most beautifying sport for women. It does wonders for the upper arms, breasts, stomach and thighs. It also strengthens the muscular system and improves coordination.

Swimming burns 200 to 600 calories an hour. You should swim at least 20 minutes twice a week.

If you sit in an office all day, hiking is an excellent sport. It tones hips, buttocks and thighs, and improves your cardiovascular system.

You'll get the most benefits from hiking if you follow some guidelines. First, avoid hiking on pavement. It's too hard on your feet and legs. Instead look for hills or mountains with well-marked dirt paths. The more interesting the area, the more pleasant the hike. Second, try to hike twice a week for at least 20 to 30 minutes each time. Third, start on paths that are flat or have only a slight incline, then work

up to steeper trails. You'll use 200 to 400 calories an hour, depending on how fast you walk and how hilly the area is. Fourth, wear a long-sleeved shirt when you hike. Otherwise you'll have a tan line around the upper arm, which looks very unattractive.

Exercising regularly makes you look better and feel better.

Jogging is an effective exercise if you go at a steady pace for at least 20 minutes.

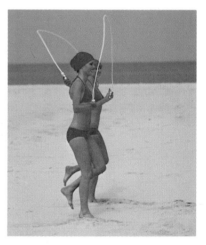

You should do it at least twice a week at first, then work up to 4 or 5 times a week. You can also increase your pace and the length of time you jog as you get in better shape. Jogging is excellent for your legs, hips, buttocks and cardiovascular system.

You'll burn 200 to 500 calories an hour.

If you aren't in good enough shape to jog each day, try taking brisk walks. This will also condition the lower body and cardiovascular system. Walk 4 times a week for at least 30 minutes. Increase your speed

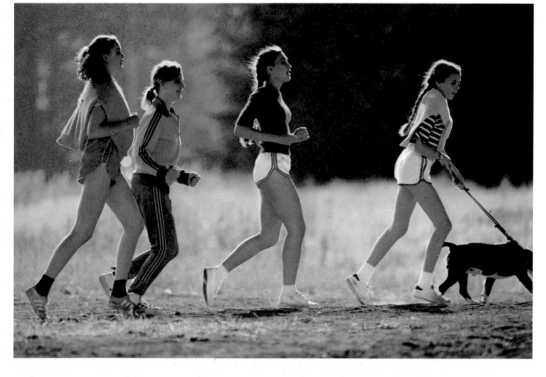

and distance as your conditioning improves. You'll burn 100 to 400 calories an hour.

Bicycling is another sport that will tone leg muscles and strengthen your heart and lungs. Even on slight inclines, you'll notice how your whole body has to work. Bicycle at least twice a week, 20 to 30 minutes each time. As with hiking, you should start off in flat areas and work up to hillier ones. You'll burn 300 to 600 calories an hour.

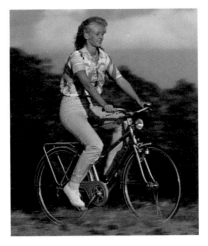

One of the easiest ways to get in shape is rope jumping. It is ideal for people who don't enjoy exercising. Rope jumping increases the heart rate and improves circulation. It doesn't matter whether you jump forward, or backward, or with your feet apart or together. The results will be the same. In the beginning, 5 minutes daily will be sufficient. You can work up to 15 minutes a day, but do so gradually. You'll use 300 to 500 calories an hour.

Tennis, especially singles, is another sport that will get you in condition quickly. The constant running tones your legs, hips, buttocks and cardiovascular system. Swinging the racket firms your arms and back.

You should play singles at least twice a week for 30 minutes. If you're playing doubles, stay on the court at least 45 minutes. You'll burn 100 to 500 calories an hour, depending on the pace of the game.

Waterproof makeup will protect your skin while you swim.

Racquetball is another sport that will get your lower body and cardiovascular system in good condition very quickly. Play at least twice a week for 30 minutes. You'll burn 200 to 500 calories an hour.

Winter sports are good exercise and fun, too. Ice skating is especially good for thighs and calves. You'll burn only 100 to 300 calories an hour.

Snow skiing is much more strenuous. It is excellent for toning legs, hips and buttocks, and for conditioning the cardiovascular system. You'll use 300 to 600 calories an hour.

Skiing has several disadvantages, however. Keep in mind that skiing is difficult to do on a regular basis. Equipment, lessons and lift fees can be very expensive.

When you start working out, you may have sore muscles. You can minimize the discomfort by ending each exercise session with a cooling-down period that involves gradually reducing the intensity of the exercise to slow down the heart rate and allow your muscles to relax. After cooling down, get into a sauna or warm bath. This will help alleviate muscle pain and stiffness.

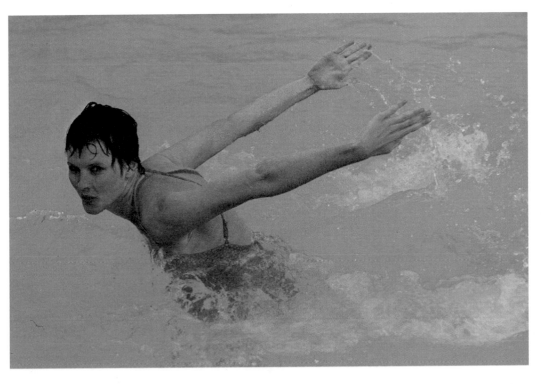

Pampering Yourself

You radiate inner beauty if you feel relaxed and good about yourself. This kind of beauty is very attractive. If you have it, you don't need to worry about whether you have a perfect face or body.

How can you achieve this serenity? How can you learn to relax, even when pressures continue to pile up? There are several techniques that can help:

If you know when you go to bed that you can't do everything on your schedule the next day, make sure to take a half hour for yourself when you wake up in the morning. Get up 30 minutes earlier if you have to. Taking the time to consciously do something that will make you feel good will be much more beneficial than 30 extra minutes of sleep.

One of the best things you can do is exercise. This will wake you up and get your circulation going.

Then take a warm shower and finish with a cold one. Afterward, try these three quick massages:

1. Put your palms on your ankles. Massage upward to the hips, using circular motions.

2. Put your hands on your calves. Gently knead the muscles. Move up your leg with circular motions until you reach your hips.

3. Put your fingertips on your chest. Do a slow massage, moving your fingertips in small circles in the direction of your heart.

Next, eat a healthful breakfast. Have something you really like. Take your time and enjoy your food. Remember that coffee is a stimulant. You'll be more relaxed if you have herbal tea without caffeine.

This routine will set you up for the entire day. You'll leave the house feeling relaxed and strong. During the remainder of the day, try not to let stress overwhelm you. If this starts to happen, stop and ask yourself, "What would I like to do for *me* now? What do I need?"

Most of the time you'll find that the answer is something that's easy to do. It may be a short walk, a phone call to a friend or just a moment of peace and quiet. You should fulfill these simple desires. The couple of minutes you spend on yourself will keep you going for hours.

There are other things you can do to energize yourself. If you're under a lot of pressure, try this yoga exercise. Lie on the floor in the fetal position.

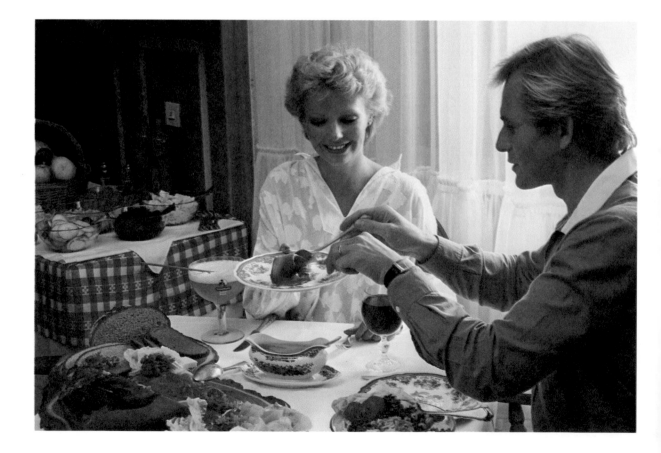

Breathe slowly and deeply for 10 minutes.

If you feel tense and rushed, purposely make yourself as pretty as possible. Renew your makeup completely.

Never take your problems to bed. Make sure you're relaxed before trying to sleep. These three breathing exercises are very helpful:

1. Lie on your back. Keep your legs together and raise them until they are straight up. Breathe in deeply as you raise your legs. Hold 3 seconds, and then bend knees into chest. As you exhale, slowly straighten legs in front of you and slowly lower them to the floor. Repeat 5 to 10 times.

Pamper yourself during the day by having a quiet meal or a long walk.

2. Stand up straight. Raise your arms over your head as you inhale. Then slowly lower your arms as you exhale. Slowly swing your arms backward as you inhale. Slowly swing them forward as you exhale. Repeat 10 to 15 times.

3. Put your hands on your

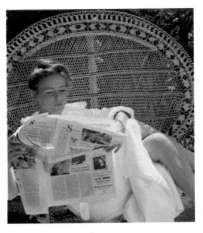

hips. Bend forward from the waist until your trunk is parallel to the floor. Bend forward more, moving your head toward your knees as you exhale. Raise your trunk back to a parallel position as you inhale. Repeat 10 to 15 times.

4. Sit upright. Close your eyes and slowly rotate your head in a circle. Start with your chin on your chest. Move your head to the right, until your right ear almost touches your right shoulder. Tilt your head straight back, until your chin points skyward. Then move your head left until your ear almost touches your left shoulder. Move your chin back to your chest. Then circle your head in the other direction. Breathe slowly and rhythmically throughout this exercise. Repeat 5 times in each direction.

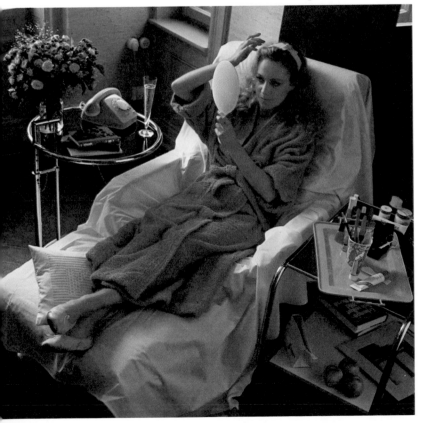

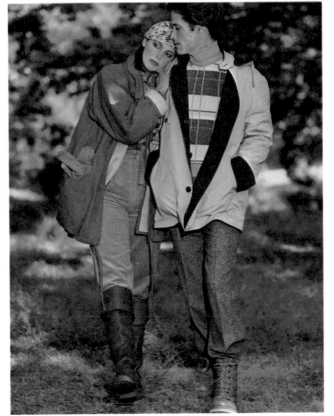

Getting Your Beauty Rest

Sleep is vital not only for good health, but for beauty. If you don't get enough sleep, you're more likely to become ill and to have problems with your skin and hair.

Sleep enables your body to eliminate waste and store energy. If you don't allow your body enough time to accomplish these tasks, you feel tired and sluggish.

Your face reflects how you feel. The skin on the rest of your body doesn't change after a sleepless night, but your face may look wan and wrinkled. This occurs because your face has several layers of fine muscle. The connective tissue between these layers usually has a lot of moisture, which makes the skin look firm and taut. When you don't get enough sleep, this tissue can lose moisture, making skin look drawn and lined.

Sometimes your face may look swollen, even after 8 hours of sleep. This may mean facial tissue is retaining too much water.

You can usually get rid of this puffiness by exercising for 5 to 10 minutes in the morning. If it hasn't disappeared by breakfast, you should see a doctor.

Don't treat this condition by taking diuretics. They make your kidneys work too hard and provide only temporary relief.

If you want to get your beauty sleep, follow these guidelines:

Take a relaxing bath first.

Air the room thoroughly before going to bed.

Make sure the room is a comfortable temperature. For most people, this is between 50F and 70F (10C and 21C).

Sleep is energizing and beautifying.

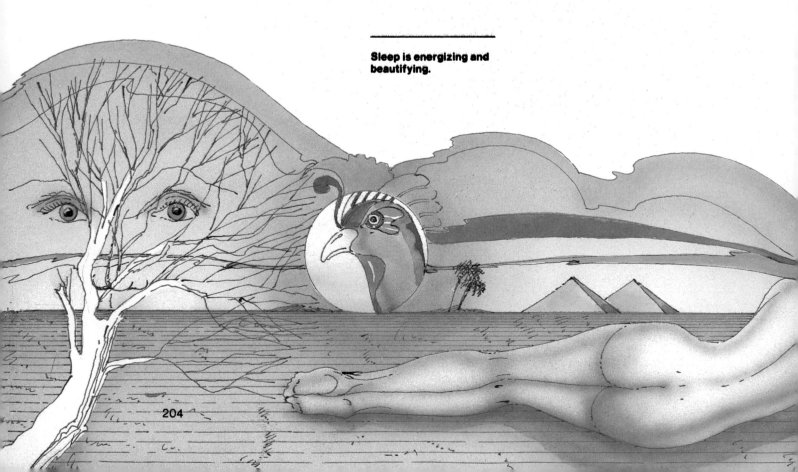

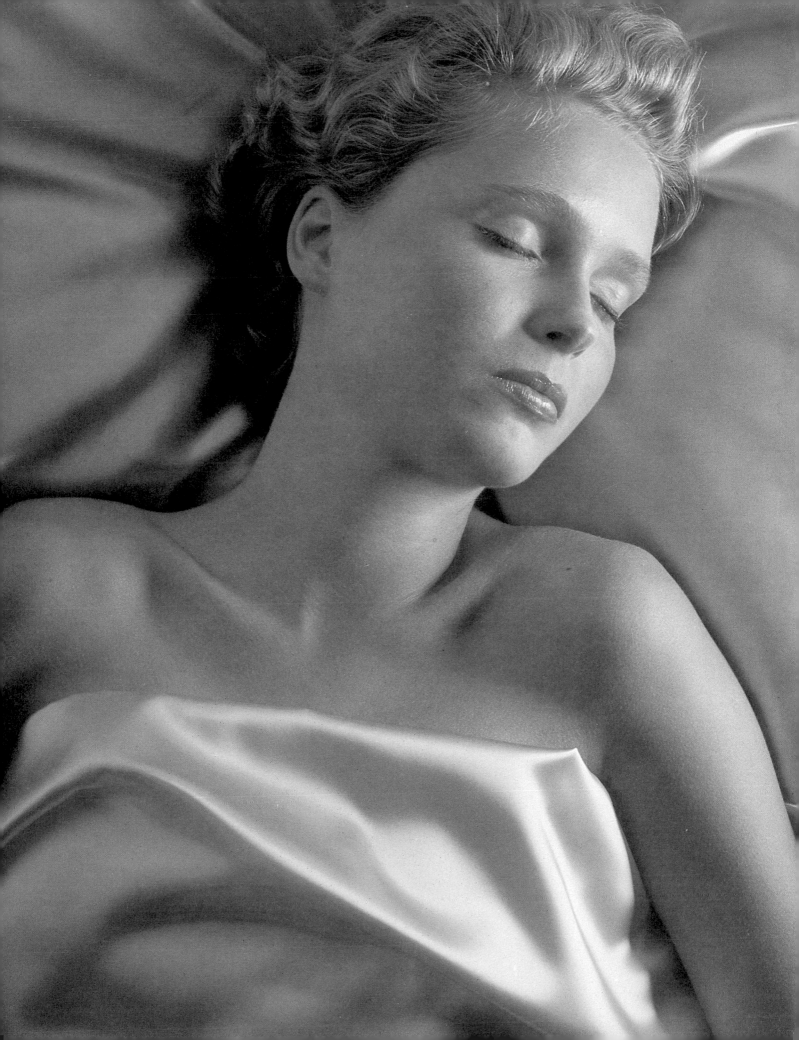

Index

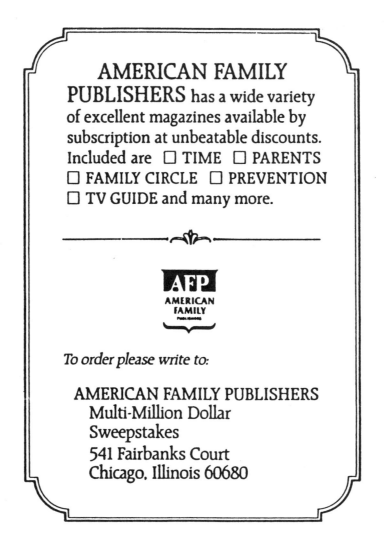